T0093331

Mental Capacity Legislation

Second Edition

Mental Capacity Legislation

Principles and Practice

Second Edition

Edited by

Rebecca Jacob
University of Cambridge and Cambridgeshire and Peterborough NHS Foundation Trust

Michael Gunn
University of Staffordshire

Anthony Holland
University of Cambridge

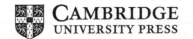

CAMBRIDGE
UNIVERSITY PRESS

CAMBRIDGE
UNIVERSITY PRESS

University Printing House, Cambridge CB2 8BS, United Kingdom

One Liberty Plaza, 20th Floor, New York, NY 10006, USA

477 Williamstown Road, Port Melbourne, VIC 3207, Australia

314–321, 3rd Floor, Plot 3, Splendor Forum, Jasola District Centre,
New Delhi – 110025, India

79 Anson Road, #06–04/06, Singapore 079906

Cambridge University Press is part of the University of Cambridge.

It furthers the University's mission by disseminating knowledge in the
pursuit of education, learning, and research at the highest international levels
of excellence.

www.cambridge.org
Information on this title: www.cambridge.org/9781108480369
DOI: 10.1017/9781108648622

First published 2019

Printed and bound in Great Britain by Clays Ltd, Elcograf S.p.A.

A catalogue record for this publication is available from the British Library.

Library of Congress Cataloging-in-Publication Data
Names: Jacob, Rebecca, editor. | Gunn, M. J. (Michael J.), editor. |
Holland, Tony, 1948- editor.
Title: Mental capacity legislation : principles and practice / edited by Rebecca
Jacob, University of Cambridge; Michael Gunn, University of Staffordshire;
Anthony Holland, University of Cambridge.
Description: Second edition. | Cambridge, United Kingdom ; New York,
NY, USA : Cambridge University Press, 2019. | Includes bibliographical
references and index.
Identifiers: LCCN 2018042529 | ISBN 9781108480369 (hardback)
Subjects: LCSH: Mental health laws–England. | Great Britain. Mental
Capacity Act 2005. | BISAC: MEDICAL / Mental Health.
Classification: LCC KD3412 .M457 2019 | DDC 346.4201/30874–dc23
LC record available at https://lccn.loc.gov/2018042529

ISBN 978-1-108-48036-9 Hardback

....

Contents

Contributors

Dr Caroline Barry
Consultant in Palliative Medicine, Norfolk and Norwich University Hospital, Norwich, UK

Dr Michael Dunn
The Ethox Centre, University of Oxford, UK

Charlotte Emmett
Associate Professor of Law, School of Law, Northumbria University, Newcastle upon Tyne, UK

Dr Elizabeth Fistein
Ethics and Law Theme Lead, School of Clinical Medicine, University of Cambridge, UK

Emeritus Professor Anthony Holland
Honorary Consultant Psychiatrist (CPFT) and Health Foundation Chair in Learning Disabilities, Cambridge Intellectual and Developmental Disabilities Research Group (CIDDRG), University of Cambridge, UK

Professor Matthew Hotopf
Vice Dean of Research, Institute of Psychiatry, Psychology and Neuroscience, King's College London, UK

Professor Julian C. Hughes
RICE Professor of Old Age Psychiatry, University of Bristol and Research Institute for the Care of Older People, Royal United Hospital, Bath, UK

Dr Rebecca Jacob
Consultant Psychiatrist, Addenbrookes Hospital, Cambridge, Cambridgeshire and Peterborough NHS Foundation Trust (CPFT) & Associate Lecturer, Department of Psychiatry, University of Cambridge, UK

Dr Annabel Price
Consultant Liaison Psychiatrist, Older People's Team, Addenbrookes Hospital, Cambridge, Cambridgeshire and Peterborough NHS Foundation Trust (CPFT), UK

Dr Benjamin Spencer
Department of Psychological Medicine, Institute of Psychiatry, Psychology and Neuroscience, King's College London, UK

Dr Susan F. Welsh
Consultant Psychiatrist in Older People's Mental Health, Fulbourn Hospital, Cambridgeshire and Peterborough NHS Foundation Trust, Cambridge, UK

Foreword

From the Foreword to the First Edition

The contrast between the underlying assumptions of the Mental Capacity Act (MCA) 2005 and the Mental Health Act (MHA)1983 (and amended in 2007) is stark. The former aims to support the patient's autonomy and permits non-consensual treatment only when the person's decision-making capacity is impaired and the intervention is in the person's 'best interests'. Even then, the person must be supported as far as possible to participate in the treatment decision. 'Best interests', though variously defined, emphasises the patient's perspective, asking, for instance, what the patient's decision would have been regarding their current predicament if their capacity had been retained. Previous preferences, wishes or values expressed by the patient should be explored, including consultation with those who know the patient well and who might be able to cast light on the question.

The MHA, on the other hand, permits involuntary treatment for those with a 'mental disorder' on the basis that the person suffers from such a disorder, and that treatment is warranted in the interests of the person's health or safety, or for the protection of others. This conceptual disparity can easily lead to confusion in psychiatric practice. The MCA applies to all patients, those with a 'mental disorder' as well as those with a 'physical disorder', but if the MHA is invoked, its provisions trump those of the MCA. If a person suffers at the same time from both a mental disorder and a physical disorder and lacks capacity, different rules pertain to the non-consensual treatment of each. If one type of disorder is a significant cause of the other, whether one of the legal regimes may be considered to cover both conditions may become a conundrum. When the question of a 'deprivation of liberty' arises, the relationship between the provisions of the MHA and the 'Deprivation of Liberty Safeguards' under the MCA seems tortuous.

The Second Edition

The second edition of this book adds detailed treatment of significant changes in the interpretation of the MCA. However, the book's orientation remains one that will help the clinician and others to apply these changes in their daily practice, based on a solid understanding of their conceptual bases.

Key areas of development include the following. The extent to which regard should be paid in the determination of 'best interests' to the incapacitous person's beliefs and values, both past and present, is moving generally in the direction of assuming stronger emphasis. The Supreme Court's 2014 decision in *Cheshire West* ('a gilded cage is still a cage') characterising situations entailing a 'deprivation of liberty' has had huge implications for practice across medicine and social care. We are presently in the midst of attempts to develop a schema for 'liberty protection safeguards' that is both practical and fit for purpose. Reconciliation of the MCA with the UN Convention on the Rights of Persons with Disabilities (UNCRPD) meets serious philosophical obstacles. An authoritative (though controversial) interpretation of Article 12 given in its *General Comment No.1* in 2014 by the UN CRPD Committee maintains that decision-making capacity should not be a basis for 'substitute decision-making', and that, in any case, such decision-making is in breach of the Convention. The problematic interfaces with the MHA remain, as in the case of deprivation of liberty provisions, which are being reviewed as an important element in a proposed reform of the MHA. End-of-life decisions involving capacity and best interests continue to present some of our thorniest ethical problems.

As I stated in the foreword to the First Edition: The clinician badly needs a helping hand in coming to terms with the implications of the MCA for his or her practice. This volume should certainly rank near the top on any list of guides to understanding this new dimension of practice.

George Szmukler
Emeritus Professor of Psychiatry and Society,
Institute of Psychiatry, Psychology and Neuroscience,
King's College London

Preface

The purpose of this book is to provide health and social care professionals' guidance when faced with challenging medico-legal dilemmas that require an understanding of the mental capacity statute. Our intention is to produce a user-friendly guide to the Mental Capacity Act 2005 (MCA) to be read in conjunction with the MCA Code of Practice.

The second edition of this book is published more than a decade after the implementation of the statutory framework of the MCA by health and social care practitioners. We have taken the opportunity to draw upon clinical experience, case law and the developing research literature regarding its use. The authors of the different chapters include both clinicians as well as medical and legal academics, chosen to ensure that practical as well as theoretical and research considerations pertaining to the statute are taken into account.

An impetus for publishing this second edition relates to emerging case law in the clinical application of the MCA, specifically of DoLS legislation. This has resulted in the Government's recently published Mental Capacity (Amendment) Bill in July 2018. The Supreme Court Judgement of *Cheshire West* attempted to clarify the definition of a deprivation of liberty by introducing an 'acid test'; 'where lack of capacity to consent to arrangements for care and treatment, continuous supervision and control, and a lack of freedom to leave are all present together, the test for deprivation of liberty is met'. Nonetheless, a degree of uncertainty continued to surround the use of the DoLS, leading to the development of the *Liberty Protection Safeguards*, discussed in some detail in chapter 4. A new and topical chapter has been introduced; the relevance of the MCA in end-of-life decision-making, focusing on supporting vulnerable and terminally ill adults when planning ahead. We have also described the growing literature and case law pertaining to applications of the MCA in hospital settings and the differences in its use in social care settings.

The MCA is not the only legislation in flux: in May 2018, *an Interim report into the Independent Review of the Mental Health Act 1983* was published highlighting, amongst many other areas, how deprivation of liberty might relate to those with mental disorder. The overlapping and differentiating aspects in the use of the Mental Health and Mental Capacity Acts are highlighted in Chapter 1.

We hope the issues covered will assist health and social care practitioners, both in gaining a better understanding of the historical background and fundamental principles underpinning mental capacity legislation, as well as in its everyday practice.

RJ
MG
AH
April 2019

Editors' Note

All the case study patients in this book are fictional but based upon the authors' collected experience of many patients with similar histories, needs and outcomes.

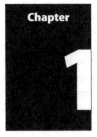

Introduction

Rebecca Jacob and Anthony Holland

The Mental Capacity Act 2005 (MCA) received Royal Assent in April 2005, coming into force during 2007 (MCA, 2005). The MCA incorporates into statute, principles and practices that had been established, through case law, over the years. It sets out how mental capacity is defined in law and how 'best interests' should be ascertained when a person lacks the requisite capacity to make the decision in question.

Prior to its introduction, clinicians and carers were in uncertain legal territory when making decisions of a social, health or financial nature for those individuals without capacity. Importantly, however, the statute is more than a solution to a recognised gap in English and Welsh Law; it is also about a culture change. It requires those in a caring and/or professional capacity to engage with a person, who may lack decision-making capacity, in a manner that involves him/her, and others important to them, in the process of decision-making. In doing so, they must have regard to past and present beliefs and values of the person concerned. The MCA, in its approach, is not so much giving power to others to make decisions, rather it is asking those who have to take a decision on behalf of another to do so in a manner that is transparent, justifiable and respectful of all issues relevant to that person. It is applicable in any situation where someone might lack capacity, including, for example, the person transiently incapacitated through excess alcohol or from a head injury requiring treatment, to people with potentially more enduring incapacity due to dementia or learning disabilities. It is therefore as relevant in intensive care as it is in social care. The MCA is both about the 'here and now', when an immediate decision may have to be made on behalf of a person lacking capacity at the present time but also about planning for the future; how individuals, whilst having capacity, can determine who can take decisions on their behalf in the event that they lose capacity through illness or injury at a later date.

Whilst it was a very significant Act of Parliament, much of what the MCA has brought into practice is what practitioners and others should have been adhering to on the basis of the developing case law. In its early development work, the Law Commission stated that people should be 'enabled and encouraged to take for themselves those decisions they are able to take'. The pivotal concept, when determining whether or not the MCA is applicable, therefore, is whether or not the person having to take the decision has the requisite decision-making capacity. This concept of 'capacity' is defined in the dictionary quite simply as 'the ability or power to do'. In a legal and/or clinical context, this might refer to an individual's ability to make a decision regarding a healthcare matter, to undertake the process of making a will or to decide where to live – in other words decisions encompassing the social, welfare and the health needs of an individual (BMA, 2018).

The second edition of this book draws upon experience gained over more than a decade of the MCA being in force. In addition to updates on recent case law, it also focuses on its application in different settings or circumstances, such as end-of-life planning and the relevance of MCA legislation in this regard. Of particular emphasis in this updated edition is the complexity of the use of the Deprivation of Liberty Safeguards (DoLS) that came into law as an addition to the MCA, followed by the development of case law in its wake. The ruling in the cases of *P* v. *Cheshire West and Chester Council* as well *as P and Q* v. *Surrey County Council* has led to a paradigm shift in our understanding of the terms 'deprivation' versus 'restriction' of liberty, and has thereby extended the circumstances when DoLS should be applied. The Supreme Court's view on this is epitomised by the phrase used by Baroness Hale in her ruling on *Cheshire West* – 'a gilded cage is still a cage'. As a result of this ruling, there has been a significant increase in the number of applications for DoLS 'standard authorisations' in England, overwhelming an already busy service. Reform is in the offing and Chapter 4 will discuss the replacement scheme for the DoLS, which instead have been termed the 'Liberty Protection Safeguards'.

This introductory chapter gives an overview of the fundamental ethical and philosophical thinking that has shaped the MCA and a brief description of its historical development and scope. It also compares and contrasts the remit of the MCA 2005 with the Mental Health Act (MHA) 1983 as amended in 2007, as there are specific situations when, arguably, either Act might be applicable. Although the Human Rights Act 1998 is not formally dealt with, either in this chapter or the book as a whole, its principles are clearly interwoven into the fabric of both Acts.

Medical ethics

It would be incomplete if a book on the MCA made no mention of the guiding principles that have come to underpin medical practice and this statute – sometimes referred to as the 'bioethical' approach. This is concerned with the framework within which a medical decision may be reached based on an individual's views, values and wishes (Harris, 1985) and also with how conflicts and dilemmas might be resolved when there are disagreements. Such conflicts may be as extreme as whether or not to start or to continue specific treatments for life-threatening illnesses. However, in essence the clinical situation is described as follows: the doctor advises as to the treatment options taking into account the patient's condition, prognosis and other relevant external factors. The patient, on due consideration, may or may not decide to accept the proposed treatment(s). The moral imperative remains with the doctor, using his/her medical expertise, to consider, after diagnosis, all the appropriate steps available to treat the medical condition and to give the patient sufficient information so that he/she can make a choice as to which treatment, if any, he/she wishes to undergo. Even though the competent patient has the absolute right to accept or refuse any of the treatments offered (except in the case of the assessment and treatment of a mental disorder where the MHA might be used to override the refusal of a competent person), barring the most exceptional circumstances, the patient cannot him/herself demand a particular treatment (Mason & Laurie, 2006).

Although a detailed discussion into the philosophical approaches that underlie the development of bioethics is beyond the scope of this book, it is appropriate to consider the theories that have influenced current medical practice. Various ethicists have put forward ideas based on different philosophical principles that have focused on either the rightness or wrongness of an act itself (deontological or Kantian theories), or the extent to which any act promotes good or even bad consequences (utilitarianism). In the former, the essential message is that we should respect an individual's right to autonomy and that each person is treated as an end in him/herself, rather than as a means to an end. Deontological theories are less concerned with the consequences or outcome of any act but rather with the factors that make it morally acceptable, and thereby uphold the integrity and beliefs of an individual. In contrast, utilitarianism highlights the moral dilemmas faced when considering the outcome of an act, that is the extent to which it leads to positive or negative consequences. This implies that the moral worth of an action is determined only by its resulting outcome. The utilitarian measure of a positive outcome, therefore, is the maximisation of happiness.

Drawing on these and other relevant philosophical theories, Beauchamp & Childress (2001) have suggested the concept of 'principlism' as a way to resolve medical ethical dilemmas. They broadly argue that the justification for our actions should be based on accepted values. They suggest that ethically appropriate conduct is determined by reference to four key principles, which are to be taken into account when reflecting on one's behaviour towards others. These include:

- the principle of respect for individual autonomy (i.e. individuals must be viewed as independent moral agents with the 'right' to choose how to live their own lives),
- the principle of beneficence (i.e. one should strive to do good where possible),
- the principle of non-maleficence (i.e. one should avoid doing harm to others), and
- the principle of justice (i.e. people should be treated fairly, although this does not necessarily equate with treating everyone equally). (Beauchamp & Childress, 2001)

The principles of beneficence and non-maleficence are not by any means new concepts and their origins go back to the Hippocratic Oath, which states:

> I will prescribe regimen for the good of my patients according to my ability and judgment and never do harm to anyone.

According to advocates of the four-principles approach, one of its advantages is that, because the principles are independent of any particular philosophical theory, theorists working in a variety of different traditions can use them. However, this approach has been criticised on the basis that it does not offer any clear way of prioritising between the principles in cases where they conflict, as they are liable to do (Savulescu, 2003). The principle of autonomy, for example, might conflict with the principle of beneficence in cases where a competent adult patient refuses to accept life-saving treatment, as will be highlighted in the next section. How then can a medical practitioner respect a patient's right, in this case to allow his life to end, whilst simultaneously striving to do good, where possible, and at least avoid doing any harm? Current ethical thinking, which is moving away from paternalistic medical practice, indicates that, regardless of the consequences of the treatment, the treatment provider must accept the decision of the recipient. Yet this may not be applicable in all cases – most importantly where a patient does not have the capacity to decide. For this reason, greater clarity is needed as to when and under what circumstances each particular principle takes precedence. Despite these limitations, the principles remain useful as a framework in which to think about moral dilemmas in medicine and the life sciences.

Autonomy versus beneficence

The central notion around which informed choice and the importance of decision-making capacity is based is the principle of autonomy. 'Autonomy' has been variously defined but, in this context, implies self-determination. People are autonomous to the extent to which they are able to control their own lives by exercising their own cognitive abilities. The acknowledgement of autonomy has served, in part, to overthrow medical paternalism and has led to the elevation of the patient from the previous position of being a recipient to being an equal partner in a treatment plan (Kirby, 1983).

In the context of the delivery of healthcare, ethicists consider respect for an individual's autonomy as morally required because it is that individual's life and well-being which are at stake in medical treatment. Respect for human dignity requires that the person him/herself should ultimately determine what his/her well-being consists of, and therefore what should or should not be done to him/her in order to achieve it. This conception of autonomy clearly implies that patients have a 'self' which is capable of determining what should or should not happen – that is, they have a set of values, the sense of what is or is not in their own interests, which may be described as the patient's 'own' values (Harris, 1985). In prioritising individual values, clinicians recognise the importance of patients' views on illness, dying, death, goals for the future, and personal relationships, when making health-care decisions. These values are highly personal and likely to result from the patient's own experience of life and his or her own reflections on that experience.

The significance of self-determination and the weight placed on autonomous choice by the courts is clearly evident in case law. As Lord Donaldson MR stated in the case of *Re T (Adult)* (1992):

> As I pointed out at the beginning of this judgement, the patient's right of choice exists whether the reasons for making that choice are rational, irrational, unknown or even non-existent. That his choice is contrary to what is to be expected of the vast majority of adults is only relevant if there are other reasons for doubting his capacity to decide.

Although it is evident that contemporary medical and legal practices broadly embrace the concept of autonomous choice of the individual, it is important to bear in mind that full autonomy and autonomous choices are ideal concepts, which we can, realistically, only attain in partial measure. This is due to the presence or not of factors that may compromise an individual's autonomy, including: difficulties in reasoning, which may be temporary or permanent; the inadequacy and uncertainties of the information available to inform choice; and fluctuations in the stability of an individual's wishes (Harris, 1985). There are also other limitations to the claims of autonomy, which include economic and financial constraints – a fair distribution of resources would clearly not allow unlimited privileges to a single individual. Personal choice must therefore be viewed in the context of the needs of 'a community' as a whole. Notwithstanding these limitations, both the ethical and legal duty lies with the healthcare professional to ensure that any impairments and limitations are minimised when initiating medical interventions.

Consent and the doctrine of necessity

It is a requirement of English Law – specifically the law pertaining to assault and battery – that consent must be obtained before any treatment or procedure involving the patient can be lawfully carried out. This is clearly expressed in a statement by Cardozo J:

> Every human being of adult years and sound mind has a right to determine what shall be done with his own body; and a surgeon who performs an operation without the patient's consent commits an assault.
> (*Schloendorff* v. *Society of New York Hospital* [1914])

Therefore, as a general rule, medical treatment, even of a minor nature, should not proceed unless the doctor has first obtained the patient's consent, which may be either expressed or implied. There are nonetheless exceptions to the above rules, which are essentially to do with situations, such as unconsciousness, where consent cannot be obtained, or where, due to a disability of the brain or mind, a person lacks the capacity to take the decision. Until the passing of the MCA, the principle that applied to treatment in these cases was that of the *necessity doctrine*. The basis of this doctrine is that, acting out of necessity in the best interests of a patient operates as an alternative defence to that of consent, which remains the preferable defence. Although the doctrine of necessity arose in relation to emergencies, in many cases this defence can be used when there is not an emergency in the ordinary sense of the word. Rather, when the usual defence is not available, that is consent, but the treatment is still considered by the treating doctor as necessary.

The application of the doctrine of necessity has been clarified by two Canadian cases where the courts clearly differentiated the overwhelming need for a particular treatment from the mere expediency of such an intervention. In the first case, *Marshall* v. *Curry*, the plaintiff sought damages against the surgeon who had removed a testicle in the course of an operation for a hernia. The surgeon stated that the removal was essential to the patient's health and life as the testicle was diseased. The court held that the removal of the testicle was therefore necessary and could not have been done at a later date. In another case, however, *Murray* v. *McMurchy*, the plaintiff succeeded in an action of battery against a doctor who had sterilised her without her consent. In this case, the doctor had discovered, during a caesarean section, that the condition of the plaintiff's uterus would have made it hazardous for her to go through another pregnancy, and he took the decision to tie the fallopian tubes. As there was no pressing medical need for the procedure to be undertaken, the court held that it would have been reasonable to postpone the procedure until after obtaining the patient's consent.

Thus urgent or expedient medical interventions are not an exception to the requirement to obtain consent. Minimum interventions to preserve life are expected in emergency situations, but in cases where there is an expectation that capacity to make a decision may improve, case law and now statute require the consideration by the healthcare professional of a delay in treatment if, on medical grounds, it is reasonable and possible to do so. The implication, therefore, prior to the MCA was that consent was imperative to all treatment; however, if that consent was not possible and the intervention was necessary, urgent and/or in the patient's best interests, the doctrine of necessity could have justified action in specific clinical situations. When applying this doctrine of necessity, it also had to be demonstrable that treatment could not have waited for the capacity of the individual to recover. It is this concept that is now codified in the MCA 2005. A surgeon working in England and Wales faced now with either of the above dilemmas, that is a patient who clearly lacked capacity due to being under a general anaesthetic, would have to follow the best interests process, unless urgent and life-saving action was required and the intervention could not wait. Thus, it is good practice for surgeons to seek their patients' views as to what they might wish to be done in the event of possible, but unexpected, clinical situations arising whilst he/she is under general anaesthetic.

In the UK, current medical and legal thinking incorporates these above bioethical approaches when resolving ethical dilemmas in the practice of healthcare delivery. This is clearly reflected not only in the MCA legislation, but also in the reform of DoLS legislation with the Mental Capacity (Amendment) Bill, July 2018 and the Interim Report into the Independent Review of the Mental Health Act (May 2018). These legislative changes go some way in addressing the principles proposed by Beauchamp & Childress (2001), of autonomy, justice, beneficence and non-maleficence.

Development of Mental Capacity Legislation

Scotland was the first country in the UK to formally enact legislation to enable substitute decision-making under particular circumstances (Adults with Incapacity (Scotland) Act (2000)). In England and Wales, the impetus for development of capacity legislature arose for a number of reasons, including the needs of professionals and carers who required guidance as to what should happen if a medical, social or financial decision needed to be made for a person who they recognised was unable to take that decision for him/herself. The case of *Re F* (1990) in particular stimulated debate about the role of the courts in medical decisions. *Re F* involved the medical sterilisation of an adult lacking mental capacity, who was sexually active and whose family were concerned about an unintended pregnancy. The court's ruling in favour of medical sterilisation stated that doctors have the power and, in certain circumstances, the duty to treat incapacitated patients provided the treatment is in their best interests. In this instance, an unplanned pregnancy was not considered to be in *F*'s best interests. Some argued, however, that *Re F* went too far in giving doctors sole responsibility and power to make unilateral decisions, based on the doctrine of necessity. The concern was that 'leaving medical decisions solely to the medical profession might imply that they were to be taken only on medical criteria' (Hoggett, 1994). It was further argued that certain decisions were so important that a court, or at least an independent forum of some sort, should make them.

The reforms put forward by the Law Commission focused on the fact that people should be enabled to take decisions for themselves but, under certain conditions and where necessary and in their best interests, someone else should be in a position to take decisions on their behalf. It was recognised that there was a wide range of decisions made by individuals, ranging from medical or dental decisions, to decisions about property and affairs, and broadly how to lead the activities of everyday life. Whilst it is, in general, appropriate for adults to take such decisions for themselves, the Law Commission highlighted that people who were vulnerable and may lack capacity should be protected against exploitation of any kind. Any legislation should be both enabling and protecting. The consultation paper *Mentally Incapacitated Adults and Decision-Making: An Overview* (Law Commission, 1991) recommended that there should be a single comprehensive piece of legislation to make new provision for people who lack mental capacity. The resultant Mental Incapacity Bill was examined by a pre-legislative scrutiny committee of the Joint Houses of Parliament before going to the floor of both Houses for due consideration. This pre-legislative committee, having taken written and oral evidence, made a number of recommendations, including changing the name to 'The Mental Capacity Act', a requirement for advocates and the need for the Act to address the complex issue of research involving people lacking the capacity to consent to inclusion in the research. The Government accepted many of the recommendations and the Mental Capacity Act (MCA) received Royal Assent on 7 April 2005 just prior to the dissolution of Parliament for the general election.

The broad aims of the Law Commission reforms are now embodied in statute. In Section 1 of the MCA 2005, the key principles that underpin the use of the Act are stated. These include:

- A person must be assumed to have capacity unless it is established that he lacks capacity.
- A person is not to be treated as unable to make a decision unless all practicable steps to help him to do so have been taken without success.

- A person is not to be treated as unable to make a decision merely because he makes an unwise decision.
- An act done or decision made, under this Act, for or on behalf of a person who lacks capacity must be done, or made, in his best interests.
- Before the act is done, or the decision made, regard must be had to whether the purpose for which it is needed can be affectively achieved in a way that is less restrictive of the person's rights and freedom of action.

Summary of the provisions of the MCA

Whilst the Code of Practice is an extremely useful guide in interpreting the provisions of the MCA 2005, a brief introduction to some of the significant changes that came about with the MCA will be presented here (Department of Constitutional Affairs, 2007). The MCA deals broadly with two specific scenarios. The first involves 'Acts in connection with care and treatment' in which an individual, lacking the capacity to make a particular decision, which it would be normal for that person to make, needs that decision to be made on his/her behalf. Secondly, it addresses the issue of how a competent individual, wishing to plan for the future in the event of later incapacity through illness or injury, might make their wishes known to, or appoint, a person to take the decision on their behalf in the event that they lack the capacity to do so for themselves. This involves the following options:

- *Lasting power of attorney (LPA)*: The MCA allows a person to appoint an attorney to act on their behalf if they should lose capacity in the future. This is not dissimilar to the previous Enduring Power of Attorney in relation to property and affairs, but the MCA also allows people to empower an attorney to make health and welfare decisions.
- *Advanced decision-making*: In addition to giving professionals and carers legal rights and obligations to ensure care is provided to those without capacity, the Act makes provisions for patients to have their own specific wishes respected even if/when they are incapacitated. This was addressed by the introduction of the 'advance decision to refuse treatment' (MCA 2005, Sections 24–26). A person can express his/her wish as to what should happen if he/she lacked the capacity to make the necessary decision. Where such advance decisions state a *wish* for some particular treatment or some other action, they must be considered but they are not necessarily legally binding as a person cannot insist on something that may be impossible when the time comes (e.g. wanting to live with someone who couldn't or doesn't wish to care for them), or may be medically inappropriate and harmful (e.g. the use of a treatment that was inappropriate for the illness in question). However, valid and applicable advance decisions to *refuse* treatment are legally binding as they represent an extension of the individual's right to refuse treatment when having capacity.

An important development was the introduction of independent mental capacity advocates (IMCAs), for those who have not appointed a lasting power of attorney and who have no others who might support them when an important decision needs to be made. The IMCA can speak on behalf of individuals, who are without family or friends, to represent their ascertainable wishes as far as these are possible to ascertain. Its purpose is to help vulnerable people who, whilst lacking capacity, require decisions to be made. These may vary from serious medical treatment to a change of residence – for example, moving to a hospital or care home. NHS bodies and local authorities have a duty to consult the IMCA in decisions involving people who have no family or friends. Of course, an IMCA, unlike a donee, *cannot* make a final decision on behalf of a patient; however, they offer independent advice to the professional bodies as to what they believe may be in patients' best interests.

During the process of reform, the Law Commission considered the need for an integrated statutory jurisdiction for making personal, welfare, healthcare and financial decisions on behalf of those lacking capacity and for resolving disputes through a new court system. The importance of this area of jurisdiction was emphasised in the setting up of the Court of Protection (CoP), which has jurisdiction relating to the whole MCA. The CoP has the remit of being the final arbiter in matters related to mental capacity, best interests principles, appointment of a lasting power of attorney and other matters in connection with interventions providing for those without capacity when specific decisions have to be made. It deals with decisions concerning property and affairs, as well as health and welfare decisions. It is particularly important in resolving complex or disputed cases. These courts are based in venues in a number of locations across England and Wales and are supported by a central administration in London. Recent data suggest that in excess of 90% of applications made to the CoP concern property and financial decisions, whilst most of the remaining applications concern health and welfare decisions on behalf of the individual lacking capacity (Alghrani *et al.*, 2016).

A new Public Guardian was created under the Act. The Public Guardian has several duties and is supported in carrying out these duties by the Office of the Public Guardian (OPG). The Public Guardian and his staff are the registering authority for lasting power of attorney and deputies. They supervise deputies appointed by the CoP and provide information to help the CoP make decisions. They also work together with other agencies, such as the police and social services, to respond to any concerns raised about the way in which an attorney or deputy is operating.

The Mental Health Act 1983 (with 2007 amendments) and the Mental Capacity Act 2005: overlapping and differentiating criteria in their application

Mental health professionals are perhaps in the unique position to observe and compare the statutes and the Code of Practice of both the MHA 1983 and the MCA 2005. In doing so, it becomes clear that these two Acts are based on different and potentially conflicting principles. The MCA 2005 respects the principle of autonomy for capable adults and sets out 'best interests' principles regarding the management of adults who lack capacity to make decisions for themselves. The use of mental health legislation in the form of the amended MHA 1983 enables treatment of a mental disorder to non-consenting patients, *whether or not the individual is capable*, a fact which has been considered by many to be discriminatory (Department of Health, 1999). The MHA is largely concerned with the circumstances in which a person with a mental disorder can be detained compulsorily for treatment of that disorder. It also sets out the processes that must be followed, and the safeguards for patients, to ensure that they are not inappropriately detained in hospital. Using a rather broad description of the purpose of the legislation, it is to ensure that people with serious mental disorders can be 'detained in the interests of his/her health or safety, or with a view to the protection of other persons' (MHA 1983).

Notwithstanding the many distinctions, there is some commonality in the defining criteria of the two acts. The Mental Capacity Act 2005 defines an individual as lacking capacity 'if at the material time he is unable to make a decision for himself in relation to a matter because of an impairment of, or disturbance in the function of, the mind or brain'; the Mental Health Act 2007 defines a mental disorder simply as 'any disorder or disability of the mind'. Other overlapping principles relate to the requirement to use the least restrictive alternative when considering care and minimising restrictions on liberty. Both statutes enable clinicians to care for patients who need healthcare interventions and who either cannot (because of incapacity) or will not, in the case of MHA 2007, agree to what is considered to be the necessary intervention. The legislation takes into account the wishes of the nearest relative and those of family or friends, and, where there is no one at hand, independent mental capacity advocates and independent mental health advocates are available to speak on behalf of the individual, although the final arbiter in terms of the action proposed is the treating clinician. The significant differences between the two Acts primarily relate to the condition for which treatment is required. Mental health legislation usually, but not always, takes precedence over mental capacity legislation when health professionals are dealing with the treatment of a mental disorder. When dealing with physical or non-psychiatric treatment in a patient without capacity, the MCA 2005 legislation is applicable.

Occasionally, however, there is debate as to which of the legal statutes apply and emerging case law suggests that in several instances, the CoP's opinion is required to provide clarity regarding the matter. *GJ* v. *the Foundation Trust* is a case in point. *GJ*, a gentleman with a diagnosis of vascular dementia, Korsakoff's (2009) syndrome due to alcohol abuse and diabetes, was detained in hospital initially under the MHA 1983 for treatment of his mental disorder. In due course, the hospital felt it would be more appropriate to treat him under mental capacity legislation, as he was primarily receiving nursing care and treatment for his diabetes. A standard authorisation for the MCA Deprivation of Liberty Safeguards (DoLS) was made on 13 August 2009 and additionally an application was made to the Court of Protection. The question posed to the courts was whether he was ineligible to be dealt with via the MCA DoLS on the grounds that his circumstances fell more properly within the scope of the MHA 1983 and that he was actively objecting to treatment. The judge resolved the dilemma by clarifying that if it were not for the treatment of the physical problem, the patient would not be detained; thus, the only reason for detention was for physical treatment. Clearly, this is not within the scope of MHA legislation. In addition, the judge held that although *GJ* could not be detained under DoLS authorisation *purely* for the treatment of his mental disorder, he could be so in order to receive care and treatment for his physical disorder (diabetes). As such, he was eligible to be deprived of his liberty and the MCA rather than MHA was the more appropriate statute in this case.

The judge also highlighted, as a general point:

> The MHA 1983 has primacy in the sense that the relevant decision makers under both the MHA 1983 and the MCA should approach the questions they have to answer relating to the application of the MHA 1983 on the basis of an assumption that an alternative solution is not available under the MCA.

It is therefore important that treating clinicians are familiar with the underlying principles of the MCA 2005 and the MHA 1983 and the different clinical situations within which each legislative framework can be applied.

Table 1.1 summarises some of the key legal, and clinical, differences between the two Acts and circumstances under which one or the other might apply (Dimond, 2008).

Table 1.1 Main clinical and legal differences between the Mental Health Act 1983 (as amended in 2007) and the Mental Capacity Act 2005

	Mental Capacity Act 2005 (MCA)	Mental Health Act 1983 (MHA)
Mental capacity	The MCA applies only to those who are unable to make specific decisions.	The MHA does not require a lack of capacity.
Mental disorder	MCA only applies to people with mental disorder who lack the capacity to make the decision in question.	The MHA only applies if the patient requires assessment and/or treatment for mental disorder as defined by the Act.
Best interests	The MCA requires that all decisions be taken in the patient's best interests.	The MHA does not require decision to be made in the best interests of the patient and detention may be required for the protection of others.
Range of treatments	MCA enables whatever care and treatment is considered to be in the best interests of the patient.	MHA only authorises the administration of treatment of Mental Disorder. However, this has a wide definition and may include feeding and basic care.
Protections available	The MCA provides protection via the Court of Protection but an application has to be made to trigger its jurisdiction.	The MHA has a wide range of protections including Mental Health Review Tribunals (MHRT) and managers with responsibilities for making applications to the MHRTs if the patient has not done so themselves.
Restraint	The MCA enables only limited restraint to be used in narrowly defined circumstances. It originally did not permit a loss of liberty within the definition of Article 5 of the Human Rights Act. This proviso was repealed in the MHA to fill the Bournewood Gap (see Chapter 4). It will, therefore, be possible for loss of liberty under the MCA where the DoLS process has been approved.	The MHA provides the legal framework within which a patient can lose his or her liberty and be restrained lawfully without any contravention of Article 5.
Decision when capacity is lost	MCA recognises several devices for ensuring that decisions are made in accordance with the wishes of a person when he or she had the requisite mental capacity, to cover situations when capacity is lost. These include advance decisions and lasting power of attorney.	The MHA, as amended, does take into account advance decisions. Clinical decisions are the responsibility of the responsible clinician; and in certain circumstances, where a person is unable or unwilling to give consent to treatment for a mental disorder, a second medical opinion must be sought before the treatment can be given.

Given the considerable areas of overlap of these two Acts, as well as the view – rapidly gaining momentum – that having a separate statute for those with a mental disorder might be considered discriminatory, current debate has focused on the pros and cons of 'fusion law' or a generic law applicable across all health and social care interventions (Holland, 2010; Szmukler & Kelly, 2016). Thus, assessment of capacity would determine an individual's right to make autonomous decisions, and best interests principles would apply if these were compromised. Northern Ireland, as well as other jurisdictions worldwide, has introduced a 'decision-making capability' mental health law, something that the Richardson's Committee mooted in 1999, when advising on reforms of the Mental Health Act 1983 (Richardson, 1999). In England and Wales, in light of government aims to ensure parity of esteem between mental and physical health as well as other concerns about the MHA, including a rise in detentions, an 'Independent Review of the Mental Health Act 1983', led by Professor Simon Wessley, is now underway (Independent Review of the Mental Health Act, 2018). It remains to be seen whether these reforms will close the gap between the delivery of physical care and that of mental healthcare.

Conclusion

The MCA is an enabling piece of statute, allowing a shift from paternalism to respecting, and supporting, the right to self-determination. However, this shift has highlighted the plight of people who might not consent to treatment, not because they do not want it, but rather because their mental disability interferes with their decision-making capacity or their ability to communicate a choice. It would clearly be unjust if such people did not receive treatment simply because they lacked the relevant capacity and could therefore not give, or withhold, valid consent. Such a situation would open the door to exploitation, neglect and abuse of vulnerable people whose actions and behaviours may be compromised due to unconsciousness, confusion or other reasons either temporary or permanent. Yet, how can this be resolved without resort to a simplistic approach that equates incapacity to the presence of a particular diagnosis or some other status, and how can those empowered to act in such situations be supported to do so in a way that still respects, as far as possible, individual choice and dignity? It is these issues that the subsequent chapters address in greater detail.

References

Adults with Incapacity (Scotland) Act (2000) London: HMSO.

Alghrani, A., Case, P. & Fanning, J. (2016) Editorial: The Mental Capacity Act 2005 – ten years on. *Medical Law Review*, 24, 311–317.

Beauchamp, T. L. & Childress, J. (2001) *Principles of Biomedical Ethics*. 5th edn. Oxford University Press.

BMA Consent to Treatment: Adults with Capacity. www.bma.org.uk/advice/ employment/ethics/medical-students-ethics- toolkit/6-consent-to-treatment-capacity (updated February 2018).

Department of Constitutional Affairs (2007) *Mental Capacity Act 2005, Code of Practice.* London: HMSO.

Department of Health (1999) *Review of the Mental Health Act 1983: Report of the Expert Committee.* London: Department of Health.

Dimond, B. (2008) *Legal Aspects of Mental Capacity.* Wiley-Blackwell.

Harris, J. (1985) *The Value of Life: An Introduction to Medical Ethics.* Routledge.

Hogget, B. (1994) Mentally incapacitated adults and decision-making: The Law Commission's Project. In: *Decision-Making and Problems of Incompetence* (ed. Grubb, A.), pp. 27–40. John Wiley & Sons.

Holland, A. J. (2010) The model law of Szmukler, Dawson and Daw – the next stage of a long campaign? *Journal of Mental Health Law* (Special Issue: (Ed. Richardson, G.), A Model Law Fusing Incapacity and Mental Health Legislation – Is It Viable; Is It Advisable? Northumbria Law Press.

The Human Rights Act 1998: Legislation.gov.uk.

Independent Review of the Mental Health Act (2018) Interim Report, www.gov.uk/government/publications/independent-review-of-the-mental-health-act-interim-report.

Kirby, M. D. (1983) Informed consent: What does it mean? *Journal of Medical Ethics*, 60, 74–75.

Law Commission (1991) *Mentally Incapacitated Adults and Decision-Making: An Overview* (Consultation Paper No. 119). HMSO.

Mason, J. K. & Laurie, G. T. (2006) *Mason and McCall Smith's Law and Medical Ethics*. 7th edn. Oxford University Press. (*When referring to this reference, we are specifically referring to chapters 1, 10 and 20, which are titled 'Medical Ethics and Medical Practice', 'Consent to Treatment', and 'Mental Health and Human Rights', respectively*).

Medical Ethics Today (2004) British Medical Association Handbook of Ethics and Law.

Mental Capacity Act (MCA) (2005) London: HMSO.

Mental Capacity (Amendment) Bill [HL] 2017–2019, July 2018.

Mental Health Act (MHA) (1983) London: HMSO.

Mental Health Act 2007: Legislation.gov.uk.

Richardson, G. (1999) Review of the Mental Health Act 1983: Report of the Expert Committee. London: Department of Health.

Savulescu, J. (2003) Festschrift Edition of the Journal of Medical Ethics in Honour of Raanan Gillon. *Journal of Medical Ethics*, 29, 265–266 (as taken from Mason and McCall Smith's Law and Medical Ethics textbook, 2006).

Szmukler, G. & Kelly, B. (2016) We should replace conventional mental health law with capacity-based law. *The British Journal of Psychiatry*, 209, 449–453.

Case law

GJ v. *The Foundation Trust and others* [2009] EWHC 2972 (Fam).

Marshall v. *Curry* [1933] Dominion Law Reports (DLR) 260. 3.

Murray v. *McMurchy* [1949].

P v. *Cheshire West and Chester Council* [2014] UKSC 19.

Re F (Mental Patient: Sterilisation) [1990] 2 AC 1.

Re T (Adult: Refusal of Medical Treatment) [1992] 4 ALL E.R. 649.

Schloendorff v. *Society of New York Hospital* [1914] 105 NE 92.

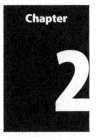

Chapter 2

The Assessment of Mental Capacity

Benjamin Spencer and Matthew Hotopf

The Mental Capacity Act (MCA) 2005 (Mental Capacity Act 2005) has had an unprecedented impact on psychiatric practice in England and Wales. The MCA originally arose out of the need to protect individuals lacking capacity in settings aside from mainstream mental health services, where the Mental Health Act 1983 (MHA) (Mental Health Act 1983) provided the dominant legal framework. However the Acts interact in complex ways (Brown *et al.*, 2013; Owen *et al.*, 2009), and increasingly it is expected that mental capacity will be assessed in the context of a decision around admission and treatment in a psychiatric hospital, even if the MHA is ultimately to be used and lack of mental capacity often may act as a gateway into the use of the MHA. Patients who are undergoing inpatient psychiatric treatment must have their authorisation of treatment carefully characterised (Care Quality Commission, 2015/2016), and the new MHA Code of Practice (Mental Health Act 2015) stresses the importance of supporting mental capacity and responding to patients' 'wishes and feelings'.

Liaison psychiatry teams, mental health services that provide psychiatric input to physical health services, continue to be called upon to assess mental capacity when a decision relates to treatment or care about a patient's general medical condition. This may include medical treatment or the setting in which care is provided or the discharge location from hospital and the consequent support (home with a package of care or residential/nursing care). However, psychiatrists are also sometimes asked to assess testamentary capacity; the capacity of a person to run their affairs; or the capacity to form a contract including marriage.

The MCA has a set of *principles* to guide its operation. These are not merely rules but helpful explanations and guidance on how to use the MCA in practice. We will refer to the principles frequently throughout the course of this chapter. Mental capacity assessments do not occur in a vacuum and the context in which they occur will alter the application of the principles of the MCA. In physical health settings, assessments are often prompted by disagreements between clinicians and their patients: most mental capacity assessments that are referred to liaison psychiatry teams for a second opinion occur in the context of a patient refusing a medical intervention that their treating team consider to be in their best medical interests (Ranjith & Hotopf, 2004; Spencer *et al.*, 2017a). Here, supporting mental capacity and overcoming communication barriers, through careful communication/arbitration, may avoid the need for a mental capacity assessment. In psychiatric care, mental capacity assessments around admission and treatment in a psychiatric hospital could determine the necessity for the use of the MHA rather than an 'informal' admission. For most of this chapter, we will focus on capacity related to treatment decisions. The same approach applies to other decisions with a caveat: some decisions retain, to an extent, common law definitions of the mental capacity test to be used (such as the *Banks* v. *Goodfellow* test for testamentary capacity, *Banks* v. *Goodfellow*). We will not cover these here.

Mental capacity is decision specific

Capacity assessments can only be made in the context of a specific decision. It would be incorrect to make a blanket statement that the person 'lacks capacity'. Individuals with dementia, learning disability and mental disorders may be perfectly capable of making some decisions, but may have impairments to make others. This is referred to as the 'functional' approach.

Examples include:

1. A patient with cognitive impairments following a head injury may be able to make decisions on how to spend money for his day-to-day needs, but lack mental capacity to determine how a large payment in compensation for the head injury should be managed.
2. A patient with dementia may be able to understand the need for taking an antibiotic, but be unable to understand the subtleties of consenting to a randomised controlled trial comparing two treatments for agitation.
3. A patient with schizophrenia lacking insight into their illness may have isolated impairments in their ability to 'use or weigh' decisions around their treatment for psychosis but be unimpaired in all other decision-making.

The functional approach enshrined in the MCA contrasts with the situation in the MHA, which uses a 'status' approach, and psychiatrists should be familiar with this distinction. Apart from certain exceptions, a patient who has been detained under the MHA can be given any treatment for a mental disorder if the approved clinician thinks it is warranted, irrespective of considerations of his or her mental capacity. This difference in approach is considered by some to be discriminatory (Szmukler & Holloway, 1998): it is as though the presence of a mental disorder of a severity warranting use of the MHA is sufficient to mean any other decision the patient makes about his or her mental healthcare is invalid. A further difference between the two laws is that whilst the MCA requires the decision maker to assess best interests, and respect advance directives, no such requirements are made in the MHA. However, there are exceptions that apply to this (namely treatment with electro-convulsive therapy), and the updated MHA Code of Practice (Mental Health Act 2015) puts great emphasis on the individual's wishes and feelings and advance directives when making treatment decisions, even if they can ultimately be overruled.

Mental capacity assessments are not risk free

A decision to embark upon an assessment of mental capacity should not be taken lightly. Being subject to an assessment of mental capacity can be humiliating and an affront to someone's dignity. Assessments are not perfect. Although the reliability of assessments when done by experts is very high (*vide infra*), there are still disagreements, and for the individual an assessment coming down one way or the other could result in substantial harm (depending on one's perspective either an affront to autonomy or negating best interests). Done thoroughly, mental capacity assessments can take up substantial time, especially when the issues are complex and attempts to support mental capacity are extensive.

Who is responsible for making the assessment?

The decision as to whether an individual does not have capacity rests with the agent responsible for implementing the decision. For medical treatment, this means the doctor responsible for the patient's care, be they surgeon, physician, psychiatrist or GP. If the decision relates to making a will or entering a contract, it is the solicitor's responsibility to assess capacity. Although all doctors should be able to assess mental capacity, there are circumstances where expert advice and guidance may be sought from professionals with specialist knowledge, for example psychiatrists or psychologists (Mental Health Act 1983). When decisions have major consequences, or there is genuine doubt about capacity, or there is disagreement – for example between a clinical team and family members – it is legitimate and desirable that mental health professionals are involved in the process, particularly as the available evidence suggests that problems with decision-making are frequently missed by non-specialists (Raymont et al., 2004). Ultimately, however, the professional responsible for delivering the treatment is also responsible for making the final decision about the person's capacity: they need to ensure that the individual's consent is valid or that when capacity is lacking they are acting in the individual's best interests.

What to consider before embarking on an assessment of mental capacity

Has the default presumption of capacity been rebutted (*principle 1*)?

The first *principle* of the Mental Capacity Act (MCA) is that mental capacity should be presumed. However, decision-making difficulties are common both in patients with psychiatric disorders (Bellhouse et al., 2003; Cairns et al., 2005a; Hindmarch et al., 2013; Owen et al., 2008, 2009; Spencer et al., 2017b) and in general medical settings (Raymont et al., 2004). When is it legitimate to rebut the default presumption of mental capacity and make an assessment? In practice, mental capacity is called into question in three main circumstances:

- When a person with a known disorder, which might impair decision-making (dementia, learning disability or severe mental disorder), faces an important decision, where consent is usually explicitly sought. This would include decisions around admission and treatment in a psychiatric hospital.
- When a person (with or without known difficulties) makes a decision which seems surprising or unwise.
- When a third party (e.g. a relative) raises concerns that the person lacks capacity.

The presumption of capacity places the onus on the agency making the assessment to demonstrate the absence of capacity, and the MCA, and related guidance, is explicit in stating that mental capacity is not to be doubted simply on the basis of an individual's appearance or diagnosis. The point of this principle is clear, and represents hard-fought battles by groups representing disabled people to ensure vulnerable and stigmatised groups have a voice in decision-making. The threshold for the burden of proof for assessing someone as lacking capacity is on the 'balance of probabilities'.

The third *principle* of the MCA states that capacity should not be called into question simply on the basis of the nature of a decision appearing to be unwise: people are at liberty to make unwise or eccentric decisions. Unless there is a more formal exposition of the mechanisms by which capacity is lacking, the final decision the individual makes is immaterial. It is not enough to argue that the decision seems unwise or 'crazy', and therefore the individual lacks capacity. However, it seems inevitable that capacity will be called into question if a person is set on making a decision which a clinical team (or other agency) feels is unreasonable.

Sometimes a capacity assessment is requested as a result of disagreement or breakdown in communication between patient and treating team. In these situations, a sensitive meeting with the patient and their family to discuss why a capacity assessment has been requested and to overcome any misconceptions or communication barriers may result in an assessment of mental capacity being avoided.

Does the decision have to be made now, have all reasonable steps been taken to help support capacity (*principle 2*)?

Has the choice been put to the patient in a straightforward way?

There are situations where a clinical team may struggle to give the patient a sufficiently clear understanding of the likely consequences of one or other course of action. Even experienced clinicians may find it difficult to convey the necessary information to a patient when the issues are emotive. Witnessing a member of the clinical team imparting information can be invaluable. It is important to ensure that clinicians do not use euphemisms when describing the consequences of various alternatives. If the patient may die if one course of action is followed, it is important to say so directly (see Box 2.1).

Box 2.1   Clarity of consequences

Occasionally, vagueness by the clinical team regarding the risks of the decision to be made can be the reason behind a request for a mental capacity assessment. For example, often life-changing decisions regarding discharge from hospital, such as to a more supportive care environment rather than the person's home, are recommended due to risk of falls or other physical health risks incurred by living alone. The clinical team may feel uncomfortable disclosing to the patient their concerns, such as the risk of having a fall if they return home, or causing a fire by leaving the gas on, or, at the extreme, being unable to look after themselves to the extent that they die in discomfort. In mental capacity assessments, such information is key to decision-making and must be disclosed clearly. Understandably, without an appreciation of the risk of death in returning home, a patient may not correctly appraise the consequence to them of their choice. A clear, but sensitive, disclosure of this information is necessary for the patient to understand the risks and benefits of the decision at hand and in doing so, he/she may avoid the need for an assessment of mental capacity.

Is there any barrier to communication: such as deafness or language difficulties, and, if so, what steps have been taken to overcome these?

The MCA makes it clear that every reasonable step should be taken to overcome communication barriers. Speech and language therapists or occupational therapists may have special skills to assist patients with communication difficulties. Signing can be used for deaf patients, and interpreters for non-English speakers. Although a patient may have reasonably good English and is usually able to communicate effectively with professionals, where English is not the first language and there is some degree of impairment caused, for example, by mild dementia, communication may be more effective when in the patient's mother tongue. Further, even patients with excellent English may not always understand colloquial or euphemistic use of language, so common in medicine (see Case study 2.1).

Family members or carers are often the best communicators with people with learning disabilities or autistic spectrum disorders and should be encouraged to participate in supporting communication. It is important to be vigilant when eliciting the support of close relatives or carers due to the risk of undue influence or coercion.

Case study 2.1 Communication problems

A young man from North Africa spoke Arabic as his first language, but also spoke English fluently. During a long admission for tuberculosis, communication had never seemed a problem. His nutritional status was poor and he had problems swallowing, so a percutaneous endoscopic gastrostomy (PEG) tube was considered. He refused this. A mental capacity assessment was requested. It transpired that he had misunderstood the doctor's description of the procedure, thinking that 'feeding you through a hole in your tummy' meant having a large mouth-like orifice in his abdominal wall. He readily consented after seeing pictures of a PEG, and having the procedure explained using an interpreter.

Enhancing capacity through treating the underlying disorder

It is obvious that when a decision has to be made very quickly in an emergency there will be less time to gather information to aid decision-making and present it to the patient. However, there are many situations when urgent capacity assessments are requested but the decision is postponed for hours or even days. Many disorders that lead to impairment of mental capacity fluctuate (e.g. delirium) or may be temporarily worsened by the current medical context (such as a person with mild cognitive impairment in pain). Treatment of these disorders may improve the patient's mental capacity and treatment must be pursued prior to an assessment of mental capacity if an assessment is needed. This not only allows more time for an assessment, but also ensures that if the person has a fluctuating level of capacity, it can be assessed when he or she is at their best. There will be 'Catch-22' situations (such as in treatment of psychiatric illness) where the only way to enhance mental capacity is to treat the illness which is the current decision for which mental capacity is being assessed. In these cases, it is important to remember that mental capacity is not static, and following treatment it may improve, and should be re-assessed accordingly. One study investigating mental capacity for psychiatric treatment in inpatients showed that around a third found to lack mental capacity for treatment had regained it either a month later or at point of discharge (Owen *et al.*, 2011).

Information necessary to set up an assessment of mental capacity

If a mental capacity assessment is to go ahead, it is necessary to know what the nature of the decision to be made is, and the following pieces of information should be assembled.

What is the exact nature of the decision which has to be made?

In general hospital settings, it is not uncommon to be asked to assess mental capacity only to find that the clinical team are remarkably vague about the decision to be made! This may reflect hurried communication on a ward round where the harassed junior doctor requesting an assessment has not understood the consultant's request, or it may arise because the clinical situation has changed, and what seemed a day earlier to be a crucial decision has now been reviewed and seems less important. However, the exact nature of the decision has to be clearly defined.

Are there a number of alternative options or only two?

Often there is simply a binary decision to be made. In other circumstances, a clinical team may be putting the choice to the patient as a simple binary one, but there might be one or more feasible alternatives. A surgical team may feel that below knee amputation is indicated for a patient with diabetic foot disease, because, radical though this treatment is, the chances of the wound healing are better. However, there may be alternatives, such as local debridement, and it is important that the risks and benefits of each of the alternatives are understood at the time the assessment is to be made. This is also relevant to determining best interests, as the MCA requires that the 'least restrictive' alternative be chosen. Remember a decision to do nothing, or no treatment, is always an option to be disclosed and discussed with the patient.

What risks or benefits are associated with each option and how good is the evidence for these?

Risks are notoriously difficult to communicate to patients, but before assessing capacity it is important to have an understanding of the likely consequences of each course of action. This is not only about risks per se, but also about the evidence regarding the impact a particular course of treatment may have on risk. For example, the consequences of a patient with diabetic ketoacidosis refusing rehydration and correction of hyperglycaemia are far better understood than those of a patient with advanced cancer not having second-line palliative chemotherapy. To refuse treatment for diabetic ketoacidosis will inevitably lead to death, and these risks are not just extreme, they are also very well understood. If the treatment proposed is little more than experimental (e.g. some forms of palliative chemotherapy), the risks of refusing treatment are marginal, but also the evidence that the treatment will lead to benefit is far less well quantified.

If the individual is refusing treatment or care, what is the history of this refusal?

Although, strictly speaking, such considerations belong to the assessment of best interests, the approach to assessment will be different depending on the seriousness of the condition and how much time the patient has had to consider the options. Simply because there has been a consistently expressed reluctance to have a procedure in the event of a deteriorating clinical condition (e.g. amputation for diabetic foot disease), this should not *necessarily* mean that mental capacity to refuse is not considered at the time when the procedure is indicated. But the refusal may be more likely to be a capable one than in a situation where a patient has had very little time to consider the options.

Is there any concern that a patient is being coerced by another person?

Although this is not strictly part of the assessment of mental capacity, there may be many kinds of pressures on patients which influence their expressed wishes and which need to be taken into account. Coercion is difficult to define and difficult to assess under such circumstances. Simply because a patient feels under some pressure might not mean that he or she is being coerced. Thus, it seems reasonable to be forthright and direct with a patient who has taken a serious overdose and who wishes to leave hospital placing herself at considerable risk, even though she may interpret the clinician as behaving coercively. Family members may persuade the patient forcibly, and it is not always clear where healthy concern stops and undue pressure starts.

However, there are relatively frequent situations where a carer or family member seems unduly protective of the patient, insists on always being present in the course of discussions and rather than appearing to facilitate the patient's decision-making, seems more likely to block discussion (see Case study 2.2). Such situations need considerable tact to be handled well, and it may be that the carer or relative needs an opportunity to express his or her views away from the ward.

Case study 2.2   Undue family influence

A 64-year-old man had a long history of type II diabetes. He had never had satisfactory control, and had run into multiple complications including renal impairment and foot disease. He had been admitted with a gangrenous sore on his foot, which failed to respond to two courses of antibiotics. The infection was spreading and he had osteomyelitis. He had appeared passive and deferred to his wife, who angrily rejected any attempt to discuss amputation with the patient. She repeatedly appeared to block such discussions and was vocal in her complaints about the hospital's treatment of her husband, as well as in her refusal that the procedure should go ahead. She further blocked attempts to assess his mental capacity. Contact was made with the patient's daughter from a previous marriage, who had a very different perspective and felt that her step-mother was furious about having to care for him and these feelings were influencing her behaviour in relation to the clinical team.

The definition of mental capacity

The two-stage test

Given that mental capacity is assumed, the MCA defines what is required to judge whether a person lacks mental capacity:

> a person lacks capacity in relation to a matter if at the material time he is unable to make a decision for himself in relation to the matter because of an impairment of, or a disturbance in the functioning of, the mind or brain.

Therefore, the MCA requires two components to be fulfilled (known as the 'two-stage test') to show lack of mental capacity:

1   The individual is 'unable to make a decision', later defined as being unable to perform one or more of these abilities (the *'functional test'*):

- The individual is unable to understand information relevant to the decision.
- The individual is unable to retain information relevant to the decision.
- The individual is unable to use or weigh information relevant to the decision.
- The individual is unable to communicate their decision.

2   Any inability is *because of* 'an impairment of, or a disturbance in the functioning of, the mind or brain' (the *'diagnostic threshold'*).

The ability to make a decision

Understanding

Clearly, ground work has to be done to define clearly the information necessary for the patient to make a decision (see above) and to ensure that the information has been properly presented to the patient. In assessing understanding, the best strategy is to ask open questions to assess the patient's current understanding, and to supplement this by providing further information in as simple a way as possible before testing again with open questions. Asking 'do you understand?' and taking the answer at face value is likely to lead to false reassurance. An example of the sort of approach we recommend is illustrated by Case study 2.3.

Case study 2.3 Assessing understanding

Assessing understanding in a 75-year-old patient with end stage renal failure and mild dementia who has refused further dialysis after an episode of fluid overload leading to pulmonary oedema.

INTERVIEWER: Can I ask what you understand is wrong with you right now?

PATIENT: I came into hospital because my breathing was bad.

INTERVIEWER: Can you say more about why it was bad?

PATIENT: They said it was my lungs, I think.

INTERVIEWER: Do you have anything else wrong with you?

PATIENT: Yes ... I have kidney failure. I have dialysis.

INTERVIEWER: I understand you want to stop the dialysis?

PATIENT: Yes.

INTERVIEWER: Could you explain why?

PATIENT: Well ... no, not really. It just seems a pain ...

INTERVIEWER: You came into hospital because you were 'fluid overloaded'. That means that your body could not get rid of the water you had been drinking and you ended up with fluid in your lungs. This happened because you had missed the last two dialysis sessions.

PATIENT: Yes. That's what they said.

INTERVIEWER: Can you repeat what I've said back to me?

PATIENT: Hm ... I came into hospital because my lungs were bad ...

INTERVIEWER: ... and?

PATIENT: ... well. Did it have something to do with the kidney problem?

INTERVIEWER: That's right. The kidney problem means that your lungs can get full of fluid if you're not having treatment.

PATIENT: I see.

INTERVIEWER: Can we just go over that again?

PATIENT: I get fluid in my lungs if I don't have the treatment.

Case study 2.3 *(cont.)*

INTERVIEWER: Yes, that's right. Can you explain what will happen to you if you stop dialysis?

PATIENT: Well ... I would be able to stay at home, and wouldn't have to keep coming to hospital!

INTERVIEWER: Yes that's right, but do you think you need dialysis?

PATIENT: They say I do, but I'm not so sure.

INTERVIEWER: Go on ...

PATIENT: Well I don't feel bad if I go for a day or two late ...

INTERVIEWER: OK, but you did end up with fluid overload this time.

PATIENT: Well, it was a lung problem.

INTERVIEWER: (after repeating information that fluid overload leads to breathing problems): Can you just repeat what I've said?

PATIENT: ... (pause). Er. Well I had a lung problem.

INTERVIEWER: OK. I'm sorry to be a pain, but I just want to go over this again. Your kidneys don't work, and the doctors have been using the dialysis machine to help your body get rid of the liquid you'd usually get rid of in your urine. If you don't have some sort of treatment for the kidney failure, your lungs fill up with fluid. You will eventually die.

PATIENT: ... hm ...

INTERVIEWER: Can you explain what I've just said?

PATIENT: Not now, dear. I'm tired.

Here the patient is making a serious decision which will considerably hasten her death. Whilst it may well be that the demands of haemodialysis are too great for her, and she may be able to make a competent decision to forgo treatment and end her life, given the knowledge of her cognitive state and the seriousness of the decision, the clinician needs to consider carefully whether she has capacity. The interview was an attempt to ascertain her knowledge of her current acute illness (pulmonary oedema) to see whether the patient was able to link this with the consequences of not having dialysis. Superficially, she had some degree of understanding, but this fluctuated over the course of a brief interview. At one point, she links her kidney disease and the pulmonary oedema; at another, she struggles with this and the interview comes to an end with her refusing to continue to discuss the dilemma she faces. On the basis of this extract from an interview, there is at least some evidence that she lacks the understanding necessary to make the decision; however, there is probably a fair amount of time over which to make an assessment, and the interviewer should return later to continue the interview.

Retaining information

The second requirement of the MCA is to ensure that the patient retains information relevant to the decision. How long does information have to be retained to make a capable decision? The Act is clear that it is not necessary to retain the information over a prolonged period of time – in other words, if a patient with mild dementia is able to engage in a conversation about a procedure and can retain the information long enough to reach a decision, it is not necessary that she retains it until the next day. The key point is that the information can be retained long enough for the person to be able to use or weigh it, and this may only be a matter of a few minutes. An example where retention may be a particular issue is in Korsakoff syndrome. The level of complexity of information to be understood can also have an impact on retention. If there is limited retention ability but the issues to be understood are complex and varied, it is possible that although full understanding for one issue can be achieved in the moment, once another issue is introduced, understanding of the original issue is lost.

Using or weighing information to make a decision

Assessing how well an individual uses or weighs information to make a decision is the most complex part of a capacity assessment. Many patients with cognitive impairments or learning disability may be deemed to lack capacity on the basis of lack of understanding or retention. Using and weighing information to make decisions is the component of a capacity assessment which is probably most often affected by psychiatric disorders, where delusions and affective states, such as depression or mania, may affect decision-making. The occasions when emotions without formal psychiatric disorders affect capacity also act on using or weighing information. It is difficult to operationalise using or weighing information, and most current debate about the nature of mental capacity focused on these issues in relation to disorders where reasoning and understanding may – at least superficially – be intact, but using or weighing information may not.

Obvious examples where using or weighing information is impaired are disorders such as mania, frontal lobe injuries or intoxication, where there may be a disturbance of impulse control, and the patient, whilst able to understand that a course of action (such as treatment refusal or forming a contract) may entail certain risks, responds to these risks in a way which seems too casual or impulsive to suggest proper using or weighing of the information. An example is Case study 2.4.

Here the patient is well able to understand the nature of the contract he is entering, and also that he has a disorder which might impair his decision-making. He appears set on a course of action, which would apparently have grave consequences for him, and his consultant psychiatrist assesses him as lacking capacity to make this decision at that point in time because he was unable to weigh information.

Case study 2.4 Weighing information in mania

A 38-year-old man with a bipolar illness is admitted compulsorily to a psychiatric unit with a manic episode. He is of well above average intelligence, and is difficult to manage. His mood is elated; he is irritable and argumentative about the need for medication. He does not have delusions, and has some insight into his condition, accepting that he is currently manic. During the course of his admission, he indicates that he has made a deal to sell his flat, which he purchased jointly with a friend some ten years before. The friend has long since moved out and has asked to buy the patient out. The consequence of the sale would leave the patient homeless and there is no evidence that he has taken any advice about the value of the property, or the legal consequences of making himself deliberately homeless.

In depression, the difficulties may relate more to a set of beliefs or cognitive distortions that lead the individual to deny him/herself crucial treatment. This may include 'temporal inabilities' around decision-making, which include viewing the future as yet to be decided and can be modifiable by current deliberations with benefits and consequences to oneself attached (Owen *et al.*, 2013). Case study 2.5 describes a familiar scenario. Here the patient is able to understand the consequences of not having her overdose treated. It is likely that her depressive cognitions, including her belief that she is a burden and that her continued existence is undesirable to her husband (despite his protestations to the contrary) and a rigid view of inevitable future suffering, lead her to struggle to use or weigh information.

Case study 2.5 Weighing information in depression

A 72-year-old woman was diagnosed with breast cancer six years before. This was apparently successfully treated, but three months ago she was diagnosed with a recurrence. The cancer was thought to be relatively slow growing and her life expectancy could have been up to two years. She presented to Accident and Emergency having taken an overdose of paracetamol. She expressed a wish to die. She understood that if the overdose was not treated, she would die. She was found to be profoundly depressed with a strong belief that she was a burden, her life was meaningless and she needed to spare her family from unnecessary suffering. She believed that her future was one of suffering; one that she had no control over and that there was no possibility of change or improvement in her circumstances.

In schizophrenia, the patient may understand the information provided by the clinician, but due to a lack of insight into their illness, this information cannot be given appropriate weight. For example, the person may understand the information a doctor provides about the need for inpatient psychiatric treatment but deny the existence of the disorder or the possibility that psychiatric treatment may be of benefit. An early definition of mental capacity from case law (*Re C (Adult: Refusal of Medical Treatment)*) included the definition that the individual had to be able to believe the information given. In observational studies, lack of insight has been found to be the symptom most associated with lack of mental capacity for psychiatric treatment in people with schizophrenia (Owen *et al.*, 2008, 2009; Spencer *et al.*, 2017b, 2018).

Communicating a decision

In most situations where an individual is unable to communicate a decision, there will be impairments of other components of the functional test of decision-making capacity. Most commonly, this will be in coma, where the patient is unable to participate at all. In acute medicine, an individual may not have had time to adapt to a disease which impairs communication. Often mastering new technologies designed to enhance communication takes time, and it may be that a patient can process the information to make a choice, but be unable to communicate it in the short window of time necessary. In these situations, not being able to communicate a decision would be grounds to indicate someone lacked capacity. However, there are extreme situations where there is sound reason to believe a patient can understand, retain, use and weigh information but is incapable of communicating a decision, despite all efforts being made to assist communication. The most pure form of this is the 'locked in' syndrome – a condition usually caused by a stroke affecting the brain stem and leading to complete muscle paralysis. Often the extra-ocular muscles are spared allowing communication by eye movement, but the most severe form renders all voluntary movement impossible and therefore, while the individual is aware and awake, he/she is entirely unable to communicate through voluntary movement.

The 'diagnostic threshold'

The second stage of the mental capacity assessment is to demonstrate that any inability found in the functional test is *because of* 'an impairment of, or a disturbance in the functioning of, the mind or brain'. Although referred to frequently as a 'diagnostic threshold', we suggest that this is a misnomer, as strictly speaking a formal diagnosis is not required to satisfy this criterion.

The threshold was introduced to protect healthy individuals, who wish to make what others might consider an eccentric decision, from having their capacity questioned. The threshold is, however, deliberately broad. Thus, although cognitive impairments and mental disorders would obviously be included, so too could temporary states of mind – intoxication, strong emotions or severe pain, which might impact upon decision-making and indeed not be recognised as formal disorders under diagnostic categories. We suggest that if the impairment or disturbance of the functioning of the mind or brain is in this category, the assessor should take particular care to explore why capacity might be impaired. Typical cases include individuals presenting to Accident and Emergency Departments following self-harm (Jacob *et al.*, 2005). Many such patients do not have a defined psychiatric disorder, and harm themselves in response to situational crises – such as breakdowns in relationships. Powerful emotions elicited by such crises can, we suggest, impair capacity, but it is prudent to be particularly careful in documenting the nature of an incapable decision when there is a relatively 'weak' impairment or disturbance of functioning of mind or brain, as opposed to 'strong' causes like dementia or psychosis.

The MCA states that assumptions should not be made on the basis of the person's appearance, condition or behaviour that he or she lacks capacity. This is a re-statement of the first *principle* of the Act (i.e. that capacity should be assumed) but goes further in making clear that decision makers should not act on prejudices related to the person's ethnic group, mode of dress, condition (e.g. Down's syndrome) or behaviour (such as talking loudly).

Differentiating between 'wishes and feelings' and decisions made with mental capacity: implications for use of the Mental Health Act

Often a person may lack mental capacity for a particular decision but still retain the ability to express 'wishes and feelings'. Many of the previous examples demonstrate this. However, the ability to express 'wishes and feelings' clearly is often conflated with intact mental capacity. Ability to express 'wishes and feelings' is a necessary component of having mental capacity but it does not demonstrate it merely in itself. Due to the MHA and the added legal safeguards around consent, differentiating between 'wishes and feelings' and decisions made with mental capacity is especially important in mental health settings – see Case studies 2.6 and 2.7.

Case study 2.6   Admission to psychiatric hospital

A 36-year-old woman with a history of schizophrenia self-presents to A&E following disengagement from her community team for eight months. She arrives at A&E with several bags packed with clothes and informs the triage nurse that she is unwell and wants to get better. On assessment, she has profound thought disorder and thought block, and only intermittently responds to direct questions with a yes/no answer. When posed to her 'do you want to come in to a mental health hospital?' she answers 'yes' but is unable to participate in further discussion or explain her reasoning.

Here, it would appear that her 'wishes and feelings' are clear, in that she wishes to be admitted to a psychiatric hospital (although the confidence we can have in this assertion is debatable). However, it is not possible to probe this decision further, especially the reasoning behind it, or her expectations, and arguably she lacks mental capacity for this decision. While a detailed discussion of the MCA/MHA interface is outside the scope of this chapter, it is worth pointing out here that it may not be possible to rely on her consent for admission to hospital, as she may not have the mental capacity to make this decision, and thus use of the MHA may need to be considered, despite admission seemingly being in concordance with her expressed 'wishes and feelings'.

Case study 2.7   Medical treatment for mental disorder

A 47-year-old man is being treated in hospital for a relapse of bipolar affective disorder. He has previously been well in the community taking olanzapine, but stopped taking it due to metabolic complications, resulting in the current admission. He is profoundly unwell and lacks mental capacity to make a decision around his treatment; however, he is clearly able to express a wish not to re-commence olanzapine.

Here, despite the patient lacking mental capacity, and although under part IV of the MHA the responsible clinician can treat without consent regardless, it is important to recognise and consider 'wishes and feelings' and the extent to which they can be accommodated as part of good clinical care. If these 'wishes and feelings' form part of a decision with mental capacity, then they must weigh very strongly when deciding on medical treatment for mental disorder under part IV of the MHA. For further reading, see the MHA Code of Practice (Mental Health Act 2015).

What does the research literature tell us about assessing mental capacity?

Laws apply to specific jurisdictions, and the English and Welsh legal definition of mental capacity differs from some used in other jurisdictions. Different components to functional tests in law imply different conceptual understandings of mental capacity. It is worth exploring the differences and similarities between our legal definition and those derived in other settings before exploring whether the wider research literature is of assistance in the assessment of capacity.

The most influential research on mental capacity comes from the US MacArthur Foundation-funded programme led by Paul Appelbaum and Thomas Grisso (Grisso & Appelbaum, 1995, 1998). This work started with an analysis of US case law, which

Table 2.1 Comparison of MCA and MacArthur definition

English and Welsh legal definition	MacArthur definition
Understand	Understand
Retain	n/a
Use or weigh	Appreciate and Reason
Express a choice	Express a choice

developed the definition of mental capacity to include four domains: the ability to *understand*, the ability to *appreciate*, the ability to *reason* and the ability to *express a choice*. The first and fourth of these are identical to the first and fourth criteria of the English and Welsh legal definition (see Table 2.1). There is no equivalent in the Grisso and Appelbaum definition of 'retention' of information; however, it could be encompassed under their heading of understanding. Appreciation and reasoning map loosely onto using or weighing information in the English and Welsh definition.

Appreciation is the ability to put information one has understood into one's own personal context, either in acknowledging the nature of the disorder for which treatment is proposed or in acknowledging the consequences of the disorder and its treatment. As such, it is close to the 'use' criterion in the MCA. A person who cannot believe the information given to him because of delusions or powerful distortions caused by affective states cannot appreciate. The sorts of questions suggested by Grisso and Appelbaum to explore appreciation include: 'what is the treatment likely to do for you?'; 'why do you think it will have that effect?' and 'why do you think your doctor has recommended this treatment for you?' (Grisso & Appelbaum, 1998).

Reasoning is the ability to manipulate information to arrive at a decision. The focus of the reasoning requirement is the way in which information is processed. Grisso and Appelbaum point out that reasoning does not imply a 'Spock-like' ideal of logic (and indeed others have suggested that Mr Spock of Star Trek would, by virtue of his unemotional disposition, have lacked capacity (Charland, 1998)). In making an assessment of reasoning, relevant factors are that the patient is: sufficiently problem focused to stick to the task, able to consider options, able to consider the consequences of those options, able to consider the likelihood and seriousness of the consequences and able to deliberate. Reasoning is therefore close to the 'weigh' criterion of the MCA. The sorts of questions which Grisso and Appelbaum suggest to assess reasoning include: 'tell me how you reached the decision to accept the recommended treatment'; 'what were the factors that were important to you in reaching the decision?' and 'how did you balance those factors?' (Grisso & Appelbaum, 1998).

For the purposes of this discussion, the importance of Grisso and Appelbaum's work is their development of a semi-structured interview, the MacCAT-T (MacArthur Competence Assessment Tool – Treatment), which takes about 15 minutes to administer, and questions the patient on each of the key underlying constructs (Grisso et al., 1997). Examples of the questions used in the interview (which can be followed by the interviewer probing further) are shown in Box 2.2. There is guidance on how to score the patient on each domain, but the MacCAT-T does not provide a single binary ('present' or 'absent') assessment of mental capacity.

Box 2.2 Sample questions from the MacCAT-T

Understanding:
After disclosure of information ask:

'now please explain in your own words what I've said about this treatment'

Appreciation:

'you might or might not decide that this is the treatment you want – we'll talk about it later. But do you think it's possible that this treatment might be of benefit to you?'

Reasoning:
After reviewing the choices the patient has made and the patient has expressed a preference:

'you think that [state patient's choice] might be best. Tell me what makes that seem better than the others'

Whilst a wide range of alternative capacity assessments have been developed, they tend mainly to focus on understanding (Bean *et al.*, 1994; Edelstein, 2000; Janofsky *et al.*, 1992; Roth *et al.*, 1982). Many provide vignettes on which the patient is questioned, but these do not allow an assessment of appreciation because the vignette applies to another person, and may well lack salience to the patient.

Reliability of capacity assessments

A review on mental capacity assessments in psychiatric patients showed that psychiatrists can, in the main, make highly reliable assessments of mental capacity (Okai *et al.*, 2007). For example, Cairns *et al.* (2005b) showed that two psychiatrists reached agreement over 90% of the time when rating a person's mental capacity for treatment using the MacCAT-T as a clinical aid. When taking agreement by chance into account, the inter-rater reliability was very high. Others have found similarly good results when using clinical aids (e.g. Bellhouse *et al.*, 2003; Raymont, 2007; Roth *et al.*, 1982). However, the picture is less encouraging when a clinician's assessment takes place without a clinical aid (e.g. Beckett & Chaplin, 2006; Cairns *et al.*, 2005b; Vollmann *et al.*, 2003), indicating how clinical practice can potentially be improved using such methods. Reliable and valid assessments of mental capacity are most likely to come about if the clinician either uses an established interview method such as the MacCAT-T, or considers each aspect of the legal definition of mental capacity in turn and is satisfied that the patient has been assessed on each criterion.

Cognitive tests and mental capacity

There is strong evidence that cognitive impairment is associated with a lack of mental capacity, but the two do not map onto each other perfectly (Marson, 2001; Spencer, 2017b). It is possible for a patient with dementia to make a capable decision despite a low score on the Mini Mental State Examination (MMSE) (Folstein *et al.*, 1975). Tests of cognitive impairment are therefore *not* a substitute for a proper mental capacity assessment, and to use them as such is against the principle of equal consideration. However, it is entirely reasonable to back up an assessment with the results of such a test. Thus, one might record that the patient has a diagnosis of dementia with a MMSE score of 17, and this cognitive impairment is evident in their inability to understand and retain information necessary to make a choice. Using the results of a cognitive assessment as an adjunct to the capacity assessment strengthens the clinical assessment.

It is important to be mindful that the impact of cognitive impairment may vary by decision to be made. There is evidence for symptom specificity with regard to the effect of individual symptoms on mental capacity: in a sample of inpatients with schizophrenia, thought disorder and cognitive impairments had the greatest effect on mental capacity to participate in research, whereas insight had the greatest effect on mental capacity for treatment (Spencer *et al.*, 2018c). This reflects that different decisions may have different cognitive demands, varying for each individual, and reinforces the importance of guidance to support understanding as much as possible and to make no assumptions beforehand regarding an individual's mental capacity.

Difficult to assess groups

Recent debate, particularly in relation to the use of a mental capacity criterion for mental health legislation, has raised the problem that mental capacity as defined in the MCA and the MacCAT-T is somehow too 'cognitive' to handle some difficult groups (e.g. Berghmans *et al.*, 2004; Breden & Vollmann, 2004; Charland, 2001). Tan, in a series of articles, has shown how patients with anorexia nervosa are apparently able to understand, appreciate and reason about their disorder, thus satisfying the MacCAT-T criteria for having mental capacity (Tan *et al.*, 2003) whilst at the same time apparently making decisions which many psychiatrists would view as incompetent. The MacCAT-T, in not addressing the impact of values, somehow misses a part of the picture. Describing a single case, Tan argued 'for Carol the paramount importance of being thin has devalued other aspects of her life, such as relationships, education, and even life itself. This new value system has made her decide that the risk of death is preferable to the prospect of gaining weight' (Tan *et al.*, 2003). If the consequences of this value system are that the patient chooses to die above gaining weight, does this truly constitute a decision made with mental capacity?

It is open to argument whether the patient's ability to use and weigh are really intact when such a belief system forces her to choose to die above gaining weight. Whilst the MacCAT-T may not be sufficiently sensitive to make these distinctions, there is an argument to say that this is a problem of measurement not a problem with the underlying construct of mental capacity. We submit that mental capacity assessments for cases in which values that could be viewed as pathological form a central tenet to the lack of ability to use or weigh are some of the most conceptually and ethically difficult cases (see Freyhagen & O'Shea, 2013, for a philosophical exploration of this area). Ultimately, for us as assessors of mental capacity, the central ethical question is whether there has been an autonomous decision, a 'true choice'. In English case law, judges have been able to make nuanced and subtle rulings in similarly vexed cases (Hotopf, 2006). A case known as 'sparkly' involved a woman with a probable personality disorder who had taken an overdose of paracetamol and was on dialysis after suffering hepatorenal syndrome, with an expectation that she would recover renal function and no longer require dialysis (*'Sparkly' Kings College Hospital NHS Foundation Trust* v. *C* [2015]). She had decided to refuse dialysis, claiming that 'she ha[d] lost and would never regain her sparkle' as a result of growing older and losing previous life status. The judge ruled that although her decision might appear unwise, she was able to use and weigh the information: *C*'s decision is certainly one that does not accord with the expectations of many in society. Indeed, others in society may consider C's decision to be unreasonable, illogical or even immoral within the context of the sanctity accorded to life by society in general. None of this, however, is evidence of a lack of capacity. Thus, she passed the functional test and evidence for the diagnostic threshold was not explored in the case.

There are inevitably some groups of patients where the psychopathology may be ambiguous and the risks surrounding a treatment decision considerable. A common example is the refusal of treatments following an overdose in patients with personality disorders or undergoing situational crises (David *et al.*, 2010; Jacob *et al.*, 2005). Here the psychopathology may appear insufficient to question someone's mental capacity, and yet the consequences of not acting may lead to the person's death. Whilst it is of some comfort that most patients who present to A&E having attempted suicide do not complete the act in the ensuing year, to assume that the person's desire to die is an indication that he lacks capacity contradicts the third *principle* of the MCA – that a person can make an unwise decision. In most such situations, though, we suggest that an argument can be made that the individual lacks capacity on the basis of strong emotions interfering or overwhelming the decision-making process.

Thresholds for capacity

Whilst the underlying psychological processes involved in capacity fall on a spectrum, the ultimate legal and clinical decision to be made is a binary one: 'does this patient have the capacity to make this decision?' Is the threshold for making this judgement the same in all situations, or is it reasonable to make adjustments depending upon the nature of the decision? When studied empirically, clinicians have been found to be risk sensitive in their assessments of mental capacity (Kim *et al.*, 2006).

Buchanan and Brock (Buchanan & Brock, 1989) suggest that the standard of capacity testing should be adjusted according to the gravity of the decision being made. According to their account, a patient who refuses life-saving treatment should have to pass a harder test of their capacity than that required had they accepted treatment. This is a risk-relative sliding scale concept of capacity testing which aims to protect patients from harm. It views capacity as functionally tied to risk, and it allows there to be a distinction between capacity to consent to treatment and capacity to refuse treatment.

Others (Cale, 1999; DeMarco, 2002; Wicclair, 1991) have argued that justifying the risk-relativity of capacity assessments on the grounds of protecting patients from harm is paternalistic and ethically unsatisfactory. Instead of tying capacity to risk, these authors tie risky decisions to high cognitive demand and argue that it is for this reason that a more stringent level of capacity be expected for patients who want to do something risky – risky decisions are just cognitively harder decisions. The authors argue that this formulation respects patient autonomy, and capacity is kept conceptually distinct from risk. The difficulty with this account is whether decisions concerning life or death (decisions usually regarded as risky) are *necessarily* cognitively harder ones, in the sense that they require a greater ability to manipulate information than decisions which are considered mundane (Buller, 2001). We can readily acknowledge that they are more profound but they may, in practical terms, be simpler decisions to make.

Another way of formulating risk relativity is to highlight that capacity determination, like any test, carries with it an error margin. According to this view, if a patient decides on something risky, then this error margin starts to become significant in a new way

(DeMarco, 2002). This is because in a risk situation to judge mistakenly that a patient *lacks* capacity results in treatment in the patient's best interests; whereas to judge mistakenly that a patient *has* capacity may result in serious harm or death which was preventable and which the patient (because s/he lacked capacity) did not freely will. Thus, the argument runs that the consequences of missing incapacity in a patient making a risky decision are particularly severe. Because of this, it is reasonable that those assessing capacity are surer about capacity when a risky decision is being made. In practice, this involves seeking more information of relevance to a capacity assessment and this may take more time (Buchanan, 2004).

Enhancing capacity and general guidance

The MCA places considerable emphasis on the importance of supporting people in making decisions. The ability of a patient to make a decision represents the match between his/her capacities (to understand, retain, use, weigh and communicate) and the demands of the task at hand. Some decisions would place considerable demands on most people and many would lack mental capacity; others place relatively slight demands upon the patient. It is desirable to do everything possible to improve the person's ability to make decisions and this can be done by either reducing the demand of the task or improving his or her capacities.

First though, it is important to stand back from the situation and not approach it as a capacity assessment. There are naturally some circumstances where a decision has to be made promptly, but many others where there is ample time, and approaching the patient simply to assess mental capacity may push the clinician and patient into opposing corners. In our experience, it is common for capacity assessments to be requested because a patient has refused treatment, and it is common for the patient to have refused treatment because he is fed up with the clinicians looking after him, and is making a legitimate if self-defeating protest. Approaching the interview in a legalistic manner is likely to backfire. Instead, the patient may need sufficient time to make a protest heard.

Capacity may fluctuate. Some causes of incapacity (such as delirium) may improve over time, and it is good practice to delay a decision until the person has had a chance to be re-assessed when his/her clinical state has improved. Similarly, capacity may be affected because the patient has just received bad news about her clinical state, and needs a period of adjustment to recover equanimity. Forcing a decision that does not need to be made instantly will reduce the individual's ability to make it.

There may be room for treating the underlying disorder of the brain or mind that is interfering with the person's ability to make decisions. An anxious person confronted with a major decision may be unable to think it through but may be helped by an anxiolytic. Similarly, severe pain may impact on decision-making capacity, and treating it will help improve the person's capacities.

Information should be given to the person in as understandable a manner as possible. Written information, which the person can digest outside of an anxiety-provoking consult-ation, may help. Diagrams, photographs and videos can all help the person better under-stand what is being proposed. Similarly, interpreters should be used if the person has difficulty understanding English.

A range of environmental measures can enhance decision-making. The conversation is best conducted in a quiet, private room where the person will be able to ask embarrassing questions without fear of being overheard. It may well be appropriate to include family members, friends or carers that the patient trusts.

There is now evidence that by using such strategies, mental capacity can improve (Jacob *et al.*, 2005; Wong *et al.*, 2000). A well-conducted capacity assessment can therefore become a therapeutic intervention.

References

Bean, G., Nishisat, S., Rector, N. A. & Glancy, G. (1994) The psychometric properties of the Competency Interview Schedule. *Canadian Journal of Psychiatry*, 39(8), 368–376.

Beckett, J. & Chaplin, R. (2006) Capacity to consent to treatment in patients with acute mania. *Psychiatric Bulletin*, 30, 419–422.

Bellhouse, J., Holland, A. J., Clare, I. C. H., Gunn, M. & Watson, P. (2003) Capacity-based mental health legislation and its impact on clinical practice: 1) admission to hospital. *Journal of Mental Health Law*, 9–23.

Berghmans, R., Dickenson, D. & Meulen, R. T. (2004) Mental capacity: In search of alternative perspectives. *Health Care Anal*, 12(4), 251–263; discussion 65–72.

Breden, T. M. & Vollmann, J. (2004) The cognitive based approach of capacity assessment in psychiatry: A philosophical critique of the MacCAT-T. *Health Care Anal*, 12(4), 273–283; discussion 65–72.

Brown, P. F., Tulloch, A. D., Mackenzie, C., Owen, G. S., Szmukler, G. & Hotopf, M. (2013) Assessments of mental capacity in psychiatric inpatients: A retrospective cohort study. *BMC Psychiatry*, 13, 115.

Buchanan, A. E. (2004) Mental capacity, legal competence and consent to treatment. *Journal of the Royal Society of Medicine*, 97(9), 415–420.

Buchanan, A. E. & Brock, D. W. (1989) *Deciding for Others: The Ethics of Surrogate Decision Making*. Cambridge University Press, 422 pp.

Buller, T. (2001) Competence and risk-relativity. *Bioethics*, 15(2), 93–109.

Cairns, R., Maddock, C., Buchanan, A., David, A. S., Hayward, P., Richardson, G., Szmukler, G. & Hotopf, M. (2005a) Reliability of mental capacity assessments in psychiatric in-patients. *British Journal of Psychiatry*, 187, 372–378.

Cairns, R., Maddock, C., Buchanan, A., David, A. S., Hayward, P., Richardson, G., Szmukler, G. & Hotopf, M. (2005b) Prevalence and predictors of mental incapacity in psychiatric in-patients. *British Journal of Psychiatry*, 187(4), 379–385.

Cale, G. S. (1999) Risk-related standards of competence: Continuing the debate over risk-related standards of competence. *Bioethics*, 13(2),131–148.

Care Quality Commission. Monitoring the Mental Health Act in 2015/2016. UK.

Charland, L. C. (1998) Is Mr Spock mentally competent? Competence to consent and emotion. *Philosophy, Psychiatry, and Psychology*, 5(1), 67–81.

Charland, L. C. (2001) Mental competence and value: The problem of normativity in the assessment of decision-making capacity. *Psychiatry, Psychology and Law*, 8(2), 135–145.

David, A. S., Hotopf, M., Moran, P., Owen, G., Szmukler, G. & Richardson, G. (2010) Mentally disordered or lacking capacity? Lessons for management of serious deliberate self harm. *British Medical Journal*, 341, c4489.

DeMarco, J. P. (2002) Competence and paternalism. *Bioethics*, 16(3), 231–245.

Edelstein, B. (2000) Challenges in the assessment of decision making capacity. *Journal of Aging Studies*, 14, 423–437.

Folstein, M. F., Folstein, S. E. & McHugh, P. R. (1975) 'Mini-mental state': A practical method for grading the cognitive state of patients for the clinician. *Journal of Psychiatric Research*, 12(3), 189–198.

Freyenhagen, F. & O'Shea, T. (2013) Hidden substance: Mental disorder as a challenge to normatively neutral accounts of autonomy. *International Journal of Law in Context*, 9(1), 53–70.

Grisso, T. & Appelbaum, P. S. (1995) MacArthur Treatment Competence Study.

Journal of the American Psychiatric Nurses Association, 1(4), 125–127.

Grisso, T. & Appelbaum, P. S. (1998) *Assessing Competence to Consent to Treatment: A Guide for Physicians and Other Health Professionals.* Oxford University Press, pp. xi, 211.

Grisso, T., Appelbaum, P. S. & Hill-Fotouhi, C. (1997) The MacCAT-T: A clinical tool to assess patients' capacities to make treatment decisions. *Psychiatric Services*, 48(11), 1415–1419.

Hindmarch, T., Hotopf, M. & Owen, G. S. (2013) Depression and decision-making capacity for treatment or research: A systematic review. *BMC Medical Ethics*, 14, 54.

Hotopf, M. (2006) Mental health law and mental capacity: Dogma and evidence. *Journal of Mental Health*, 15(1), 1–16.

Jacob, R., Clare, I. C., Holland, A., Watson, P. C., Maimaris, C. & Gunn, M. (2005) Self-harm, capacity, and refusal of treatment: Implications for emergency medical practice – prospective observational study. *Emergency Medicine Journal*, 22(11), 799–802.

Janofsky, J. S., McCarthy, R. J. & Folstein, M. F. (1992) The Hopkins Competency Assessment Test: A brief method for evaluating patients' capacity to give informed consent. *Hospital and Community Psychiatry*, 43(2), 132–136.

Kim, S. Y., Caine, E. D., Swan, J. G. & Appelbaum, P. S. (2006) Do clinicians follow a risk-sensitive model of capacity-determination? An experimental video survey. *Psychosomatics*, 47(4), 325–329.

Marson, D. C. (2001) Loss of competency in Alzheimer's disease: Conceptual and psychometric approaches. *International Journal of Law and Psychiatry*, 24(2–3), 267–283.

Mental Capacity Act (MCA) (2005) London: HMSO.

Mental Health Act (MHA) (1983) London: HMSO.

Mental Health Act (MHA) (2015) Code of Practice, published pursuant to Section 118 of the Mental Health Act 1983. London: HMSO.

Okai, D., Owen, G., McGuire, H., Singh, S., Churchill, R. & Hotopf, M. (2007) Mental capacity in psychiatric patients: Systematic review. *British Journal of Psychiatry*, 191, 291–297.

Owen, G. S., Richardson, G., David, A. S., Szmukler, G., Hayward, P. & Hotopf, M. (2008) Mental capacity to make decisions on treatment in people admitted to psychiatric hospitals: Cross sectional study. *British Medical Journal*, 337, 448.

Owen, G. S., Szmukler, G., Richardson, G., David, A. S., Hayward, P., Rucker, J., et al. (2009) Mental capacity and psychiatric in-patients: Implications for the new mental health law in England and Wales. *British Journal of Psychiatry*, 195(3), 257–263.

Owen, G. S., Ster, I. C., David, A. S., Szmukler, G., Hayward, P., Richardson, G., et al. (2011) Regaining mental capacity for treatment decisions following psychiatric admission: A clinico-ethical study. *Psychological Medicine*, 41(1), 119–128.

Owen, G. S., Freyenhagen, F., Hotopf, M. & Martin, W. (2013) Temporal inabilities and decision-making capacity in depression. *Phenomenology and the Cognitive Sciences*, 14(1), 163–182.

Ranjith, G. & Hotopf, M. (2004) 'Refusing treatment – please see': An analysis of capacity assessments carried out by a liaison psychiatry service. *Journal of the Royal Society of Medicine*, 97(10), 480–482.

Raymont, V., Bingley, W., Buchanan, A., David, A. S., Hayward, P., Wessely, S., et al. (2004) Prevalence of mental incapacity in medical inpatients and associated risk factors: Cross-sectional study. *Lancet*, 364(9443), 1421–1427.

Raymont, V., Buchanan, A., David, A. S., Hayward, P., Wessely, S. & Hotopf, M. (2007) The inter-rater reliability of mental capacity assessments. *International Journal of Law and Psychiatry*, 30(2), 112–117.

Roth, L. H., Lidz, C. W., Meisel, A., Soloff, P. H., Kaufman, K. & Spiker, D. G., et al. (1982) Competency to decide about treatment or research: An overview of some empirical data. *International Journal of Law and Psychiatry*, 5(1), 29–50.

Spencer, B. W. J., Gergel, T., Hotopf, M. & Owen, G. (2018c) Unwell in hospital but not incapable: Dissociation of decision-making capacity for treatment and research in inpatients with schizophrenia and related psychoses. A cross sectional study. *British Journal of Psychiatry*, 213(2), 484–489.

Spencer, B. W. J., Wilson, G., Okon-Rocha, E., Owen, G. S. & Wilson, J. C. (2017a) Capacity in vacuo: An audit of decision-making capacity assessments in a liaison psychiatry service. *BJPsych Bulletin*, 41(1), 7–11.

Spencer, B. W. J., Shields, G., Gergel, T., Hotopf, M. & Owen, G. S. (2017b) Diversity or disarray? A systematic review of decision-making capacity for treatment and research in schizophrenia and other non-affective psychoses. *Psychological Medicine*, 47(11), 1906–1922.

Szmukler, G. & Holloway, F. G. (1998) Mental health legislation is now a harmful anachronism. *Psychiatric Bulletin*, 22, 662–665.

Tan, J., Hope, T. & Stewart, A. (2003) Competence to refuse treatment in anorexia nervosa. *International Journal of Law and Psychiatry*, 26(6), 697–707.

Vollmann, J., Bauer, A., Danker-Hopfe, H. & Helmchen, H. (2003) Competence of mentally ill patients: A comparative empirical study. *Psychological Medicine*, 33(8), 1463–1471.

Wicclair, M. R. (1991) Patient decision-making capacity and risk. *Bioethics*, 5(2), 91–104.

Wong, J. G., Clare, I. C. H., Holland, A. J., *et al.* (2000) The capacity of people with a 'mental disability' to make a health care decision. *Psychological Medicine*, 30, 295–306.

Case law

Banks v. *Goodfellow* 1870 LR 5QB 549.

Re C (Adult: Refusal of Medical Treatment) 1994 1 All ER 819.

'Sparkly' Kings College Hospital NHS Foundation Trust v. *C* [2015] 2015 EWCOP 80.

Best Interests

Charlotte Emmett and Julian C. Hughes

At the heart of the Mental Capacity Act (MCA) lies 'best interests'. As we have seen, one of the key principles of the Act is that, if someone lacks capacity, any decision made on the person's behalf must be in his or her best interests.

Section 1: Principle 5

'An act done, or decision made, under this Act for or on behalf of a person who lacks capacity must be done, or made, in his best interests.'

Section 4 of the MCA concerns best interests and sets out certain steps that must be followed in order to determine a person's best interests. Before considering these steps, however, it is worth pausing to reflect on just what the notion of 'best interests' might mean. This should help us to understand the approach taken in the Act.

What are 'best interests'?

Whereas the MCA defines what it means by a 'lack of capacity', it does not define 'best interests'. The Code of Practice gives some reasons why this is so.

'Best interests' is not defined in the Act

'because so many different types of decisions and actions are covered by the Act, and so many different people and circumstances are affected by it' (Code of Practice, paragraph 5.5).

The implication is that trying to define 'best interests' would be a hopeless task. Clearly, the notion implies whatever is best for the person. But it is not immediately apparent how this should be determined. For one thing, it might depend on the perspective from which 'what is best' is judged. We can easily imagine a scenario in which what the person thinks is best might differ from what the person's family might think is best (say, for instance, the person has cancer and has been offered chemotherapy that will not cure the disease but will prolong life by a matter of a few months). We can also imagine a patient and a doctor having different views about what might be best (perhaps, in some other form of cancer, there are good grounds for thinking that radical surgery would be curative, so the doctors are encouraging it). In both these cases, we can imagine the family and the doctor putting forward their respective views showing genuine concern, stating that it would, in the former case, be best if the person were to accept the palliative chemotherapy and, in the latter, curative surgery. From a neutral perspective, it is simply not possible to say who is right and who is wrong in a definitive way. There may be objective facts supporting the arguments about what is best (e.g. 'the cure rate from this form of surgery is 80%'), but there are also subjective arguments (e.g. 'I just cannot face the prospect of mutilating surgery which will take months to get over'). All sorts of other arguments might come into the equation, but in the end a particular perspective must be taken: a particular person's view must hold sway.

It is important to appreciate that the notion of best interests under the MCA only comes into play when a person is judged to lack the capacity to make a particular decision. So although different parties may have conflicting views about what would be in the incapacitated person's best interests – including the incapacitated person themselves – it is the 'decision maker', the person or body charged with carrying out the act or making the decision, who has the final say. Nevertheless, when arriving at that decision the views of the incapacitated person, whom the action or decision concerns, are a significant factor. Lady Justice Hale stated as much in the Supreme Court case of *Aintree* v. *James* in 2013 when the Court had to decide whether continuing to provide life-sustaining treatment to Mr James, who was in a minimally conscious state, was in his best interests:

> insofar as it is possible to ascertain the patient's wishes and feelings, his beliefs and values or the things which were important to him, it is those which should be taken into account because they are a component in making the choice which is right for him as an individual human being.
>
> (Lady Justice Hale, *Aintree* v. *James*)

Accordingly, the person concerning whom acts are being done or decisions made should be centre stage: his or her views should hold significant sway. Therefore:

- anyone making a decision for someone who lacks capacity should do so from the perspective of that person;
- a key question will always be: what would the person him or herself have decided under these circumstances?

In this sense, the MCA best interests test contains a strong element of 'substituted judgement'. In other words, when determining the best interests of someone who lacks capacity, you should set aside your own feelings, beliefs and values, and substitute their wishes and feelings, their beliefs and values, along with all the other factors they would be likely to consider had they had capacity. However, adopting a strict substituted judgement approach requires the decision maker to give effect to those known wishes and feelings – and this is not necessarily the case when determining best interests under the MCA. As Lady Hale confirmed in *Aintree* at paragraph 24: 'This is ... still a "best interests" rather than a "substituted judgement" test, but one which accepts that the preferences of the person concerned are an important component in deciding where his best interests lie.' And later, at paragraph 45: 'The purpose of the best interests test is to consider matters from the patient's point of view. That is not to say that his wishes must prevail, any more than those of a fully capable patient must prevail. We cannot always have what we want.'

Accordingly, the wishes and beliefs of the incapacitated person are just one factor, albeit a significant factor, for a decision maker to weigh in the balance when arriving at an objective judgement as to where a person's best interests lie.

Given that we set great store on the possibility of autonomous decision-making – in other words we believe that people should, if possible, be at liberty to make their own decisions – emphasising an incapacitated person's own past and present wishes, values and beliefs in the best interests determination seems to be an appropriate approach, precisely because any outcome would aim to reflect what is 'right' for that person as an 'individual human being'.

It is also an approach that is more in keeping with the current international disability rights agenda, in particular the *UN Convention on the Rights of Persons with Disabilities* (CRPD), which the UK ratified in 2009. In doing so, the Government committed itself to promoting and protecting the full enjoyment of human rights by disabled people, ensuring they have legal capacity on a par with those without disability. Amongst its many provisions, the CRPD requires contracting states to 'respect the rights, will and preferences of the person' when setting out measures relating to the exercise of legal capacity (Article 12(4)). Strictly interpreted, this means that any surrogate decision-making model with the potential to override the known wishes of an incapacitated person is, by its very nature, CRPD non-compliant. This causes particular difficulties for the best interests decision-making model of the MCA.

The Law Commission attempted to address these concerns during its review of Mental Capacity and Deprivation of Liberty Safeguards in 2017 (Law Commission, 2017). In its draft Bill, the Commission proposed to amend Section 4 of the MCA, to impose a positive duty on decision makers to ascertain, so far as is reasonably practicable: (a) the person's past and present wishes and feelings, (b) the beliefs and values which would be likely to influence his decision if he had capacity and (c) any other factors that he would be likely to consider if he were able to do so. When weighing up best interests, decision makers would be required to give particular weight to any wishes or feelings ascertained, thereby elevating the status of the incapacitated person's wishes and feelings above the other factors in the Section 4 checklist. Perhaps regrettably, the Government decided not to take up this particular proposal and the Mental Capacity (Amendment) Bill, published on 4 July 2018 made no mention of giving particular weight to *P*'s wishes and feelings in any best-interests determination. It remains to be seen whether this issue will be revisited during the Bill's passage through Parliament and further amendments made. If enacted, it would signal a step towards support for a more CRPD-compliant decision-making model, reflecting a more person-centred approach and one that is increasingly evident in the courts (Ruck-Keene & Auckland, 2015).

The difficulty associated with prioritising an individual's past wishes and feelings is that we may have little idea what the person would have wanted under the precise circumstances that apply at the time. (Of course, our certainty increases if the person has a lasting power of attorney (LPA) or if they have made an advance statement of treatment preferences, but even under these circumstances we cannot know for sure.) Equally, an individual may be profoundly disabled and may have lacked capacity from birth, so that a strong substituted judgement approach, which prioritises a person's wishes, feelings and beliefs, would be neither practical nor possible. In these circumstances, it might be better to draw up a balance sheet of objective factors, adopting the 'reasonable person's' view of what is best, setting out the advantages and disadvantages of any proposal and drawing widely from the views of family and carers (as the court did in *Re AK (Gift Application)* [2014]).

Hence, in thinking about best interests we end up with several different strands: there are not only objective considerations, but also subjective opinions; there is a strong element of substituted judgement, but this is difficult to work out and know with any certainty; and, meanwhile, it might yet be that a 'balance-sheet' of objective factors would provide the best way to take things forward in the absence of definite evidence concerning what the person would have wanted. It can reasonably be argued that the MCA, by not defining 'best interests', allows room for all of these factors to be taken into consideration. It does this by providing 'a checklist of common factors that must always be considered by anyone who needs to decide what is in the best interests of a person who lacks capacity in any particular situation' (Code of Practice, paragraph 5.6). But the Code goes on to warn:

> This checklist is only the starting point: in many cases, extra factors will need to be considered.
> (Code of Practice, paragraph 5.6)

The checklist

The MCA sets out steps that should be taken to determine a person's best interests. In the Code of Practice, these steps have become known as the checklist and they can be summarised as follows:

- Avoid discrimination
- Identify all relevant circumstances
- Assess whether the person might regain capacity
- Encourage participation
- Do not be motivated by a desire to bring about the person's death
- Find out the person's views
- Consult others
- Avoid restricting the person's rights
- Take all of the above into account.

We shall now take each of these steps in turn to discuss and expand upon them. But before we do, it must also be remembered that when acting or deciding in someone's best interests, 'regard' should be had to the principle of minimum interference at Section 1(6).[1] Therefore, whatever the final decision or act being proposed, some thought must be given to whether it is the least restrictive of a person's rights and freedoms of action and is a proportionate response in all the circumstances – or indeed to whether there is a need to intervene at all.

Avoiding discrimination

Just as, in Section 2 of the MCA, age, appearance, condition or behaviour cannot be taken, without further justification, to mean that the person lacks capacity, so too in Section 4(1) it is made plain that these same factors should not be used to determine what is in someone's best interests. This is sometimes referred to as the 'principle of equal consideration'. The aim is to avoid discrimination against people who lack capacity, because there is no reason for them to be treated less favourably than anyone else.

The Code spells out (in paragraph 5.17) that 'appearance' includes a broad range of physical attributes, 'including skin colour, mode of dress and any visible medical problems, disfiguring scars or other disabilities'. 'Condition' not only refers to physical and intellectual conditions, as well as age-related illnesses, but also to 'temporary conditions (such as drunkenness or unconsciousness)'. Aspects of behaviour include anything that might be unusual to others, such as 'talking too loudly or laughing inappropriately'.

Case study 3.1   Mrs Able and non-discrimination

Mrs Able, a 76-year-old widow who was admitted after having had a large left-sided cerebral haemorrhage, which resulted in a dense paralysis affecting her right side. She is currently fluctuating in and out of consciousness, already has evidence of marked speech problems, cannot swallow, dribbles and is incontinent. A decision has to be made about her continuing requirements for artificial nutrition and hydration. Since she lacks capacity to decide for herself, a decision will need to be made in her best interests.

The importance of Section 4(1) of the MCA is that, in circumstances such as Case study 3.1, Mrs Able's age, her stroke and her general dependence are not good enough grounds for presuming that she requires a best interests decision to be made for her. It is still incumbent upon the medical team looking after her to go through the checklist in order to determine what might be best for her. If called upon for advice, psychiatrists might need to remind those making decisions of this 'principle of equal consideration'.

All relevant circumstances

The Code very sensibly states:

> Because every case – and every decision – is different, the law can't set out all the factors that will need to be taken into account in working out someone's best interests.
>
> (paragraph 5.13)

Nevertheless, the Act itself (in Section 4(2)) initially seems quite uncompromising:

> The person making the determination must consider all the relevant circumstances.

This is made less stringent when 'relevant circumstances' is defined in Section 4(11) as those:

(a) of which the person making the determination is aware, and

(b) which it would be reasonable to regard as relevant.

The word 'reasonable' appears in a number of places in the MCA. When it does, the effect is certainly not to excuse the person (in this case determining best interests) from making efforts to ascertain as many facts as possible, but it does acknowledge that there is a limit to what can reasonably be expected.

Thus, if the best interests decision concerns treatment, it would be reasonable for the doctor to consider the clinical indications, the potential benefits and burdens of the treatment and the likely outcome for the patient of receiving or not receiving it. The more serious the treatment or condition, the more reasonable it would be to consider these issues more broadly. For a major medical condition, it might be reasonable to bring into consideration life expectancy, but this would not be a reasonable matter to consider if the treatment were relatively minor. Importantly, considerations are not simply confined to medical issues; it would be reasonable to look at the patient's best interests in the broadest sense, considering the wider social and psychological impact of any proposed treatment too.[2] Similarly, if the decision were a social matter, what might be considered reasonably relevant would depend on the nature of the decision and would be broadly drawn.

Whilst the considerations listed in Section 4 of the MCA are not ranked in order of importance, the weight attached to a particular fact, or factors, will vary from case to case. For example, in one instance a person's known cultural background or religious beliefs might be so significant, or of such 'magnetic importance', that they will have a decisive influence on the outcome of the decision, whilst in another case they may carry little or no weight at all.[3]

In an interesting case heard in 2009, it was considered to be in the best interests of an 80-year-old Nigerian woman to be returned to her country of origin to die, in spite of known issues of risk associated with travelling and the resulting quality of care. Justice Hedley summed up his reasoning as follows:

> It is an integral part of the concept of best interests when dealing with a person of this age that the court recognises the imminent possibility of death and the importance of making arrangements so as to secure that the experience of death may be in the context which is most congenial and peaceful that can be devised. Also implicit in the concept of best interests is the importance of country and culture of origin and the whereabouts of family. They will often take precedence over, for example, the question of risk avoidance or the exact quality of care that may be available.[4]

Case study 3.2   Relevant circumstances and social interventions

Miss Plum is a spinster who lives alone but now has dementia. Providing a support worker to visit and sometimes take her out would require consideration of her wishes and feelings, as described in the details of the checklist for determining her best interests. It would be relevant that Miss Plum used to enjoy visits to the shops with friends.

If, however, the decision were to do with moving Miss Plum into long-term care, there would be a wider range of issues to consider: the reasons for the move (whether to do with safety or ill health), Miss Plum's attitude to socialising, the geographical location of the home in question, her previous interests and whether the home might be able to accommodate or encourage them, the ease with which her remaining family and friends might be able to visit and so on.

Geographical location is an example of a factor not overtly mentioned in the checklist, but it would be a factor that it was 'reasonable to regard as relevant' in making this particular decision and it would, therefore, fall under the description of Section 4(2) as one of the 'relevant circumstances' that *must* be considered. In fact, for Miss Plum, remaining in a specific location might be an emotional component associated with her living arrangements which rates extremely highly, and be of such 'magnetic importance' that it determines the outcome of any decision made.[5]

Regaining capacity

Section 4(3) of the MCA states that the person determining best interests must consider whether it is likely that the person who lacks capacity might regain it in order to make the decision in question and, if so, when that might be. The gist of this section is that if a decision can be deferred, it should be. In a real emergency (e.g. to do with medical treatment, or to do with providing emergency accommodation), by definition, the decision cannot be put off and the duty is to act. But it may be that there is time to spare and, indeed, the person may develop the necessary skills to make the decision with the right support. The Code lists examples of factors that may indicate the person might regain or develop the appropriate capacity in the future (Code of Practice, paragraph 5.28):

- where the cause of the lack of capacity can be treated;
- where the lack of capacity is likely to decrease in time (e.g. if caused by medication or alcohol, or sudden shock);

- where there is the possibility of new learning, for instance where a person with learning disability acquires new skills or increases understanding by new experiences;
- where the person has a condition that causes capacity to come and go (as in some mental illnesses);
- where the person has been unable to communicate but learns a new way to do so.

Case study 3.3   Mr Daley and the return of capacity

Mr Daley has a history of bipolar affective disorder and is currently manic. His speech shows flight of ideas. He is unable to concentrate on any particular subject for more than a few seconds and is constantly on the move. His relapse has been precipitated, as in the past, by his lack of compliance with medication. But he has accepted hospital admission and is now taking a neuroleptic drug again. There is evidence that his mania is starting to settle. At this point, his sister arrives with the news that Mr Daley has just inherited a large sum of money from a maiden aunt. He wishes to invest the money immediately in stocks and shares, but he is assessed as lacking capacity to make such a decision. Instead, it is decided that a decision about what to do with the money in the longer term does not have to be made immediately, but can be put off until he has regained the capacity to make the required decisions.

Encourage participation

Just as it states in the third principle of the MCA that 'all practicable steps' must be taken to help a person to make decisions for him/herself, so too, in connection with best interests, it states that 'so far as reasonably practicable' the person deciding on best interests must:

> permit and encourage the person to participate, or to improve his ability to participate, as fully as possible in any act done for him and any decision affecting him.

(Section 4(4))

It is important to realise that just because someone lacks capacity, it does not necessarily mean they cannot join in decisions that affect them. For instance, a woman with dementia might be judged to lack the capacity to manage her finances, but she might still be able to agree that she needs to go shopping to buy some new clothes and she might still enjoy the experience of doing so. The MCA encourages this sort of participation.

Taking every practicable means to help the person participate might entail fairly simple measures to ensure the person can hear and see whatever is required. There should certainly be attempts to explain matters in terms they will be able to understand. It might be that there is someone close to the person (a friend or relative) who might be able to convey the sort of information that needs to be considered in order to decide what will be best. The Code gives these examples (but they are not intended to be exhaustive):

- use simple language and/or illustrations or photographs to help the person understand the options;
- ask the person about the decision at a time and place where he or she is likely to feel relaxed;
- the information should be broken down into easy-to-understand points;
- specialist interpreters or signers might be required to aid communication (Code of Practice, paragraph 5.24).

The words 'reasonably practicable' recognise that in emergency situations for example, it would not be appropriate, nor indeed in a person's best interests, to delay acting in order to ensure participation.

Case study 3.4 Joining in decisions

Maria, who is 29 years old, has a moderate degree of learning disability and has lived for three years in a house with two other people with learning disabilities. Supportive care is provided throughout the day and night by dedicated staff. Although it is mostly a settled home, every now and again Maria becomes quite agitated and verbally hostile towards her carers and the other two people with whom she lives. These episodes are worrying for all concerned, but they tend to settle fairly quickly.

The lease of the property in which they live is coming to an end and they are being asked to move. It is not thought that Maria or the people with whom she lives have capacity to decide where to live next. An advocate service* has been employed to talk with Maria, her family and her co-residents to establish what might be best for them. They start by meeting to discuss where might be a good place to live. They have been encouraged to draw pictures of the type of place they might like to live in. They look at pictures in magazines and newspapers of different houses. They visit different places in the city. They have talked alone to the advocate about the pros and cons of living with other people and about with whom they might wish to live. This included help to write their thoughts down and they have had a chance to discuss their feelings again at a later meeting. All of the work on the decision has been collated in a big book which they are able to keep and look at when they want. With Maria's permission, the advocate has also talked to Maria's mother to find out her thoughts. By these means, Maria has been encouraged to participate in the decision and the advocate is able to represent her views with her at meetings with her social worker.

(*This is not an example of using an independent mental capacity advocate as laid down in Sections 35–41 of the MCA, because in this case Maria does have a mother. Nonetheless, it was felt to be good practice to have an independent voice speaking with and for Maria.)

Life-sustaining treatment

At the time the MCA was passed in April 2005, there was a lot of concern that it would allow or encourage euthanasia – if not active euthanasia, then passively by omission. Section 4(5) of the MCA goes some way towards settling these concerns:

> Where the determination [of best interests] relates to life-sustaining treatment [the person making the decision] must not, in considering whether the treatment is in the best interests of the person concerned, be motivated by a desire to bring about his death.

Towards the end of the MCA, the point is further hammered home:

Section 62: Scope of the Act

For the avoidance of doubt, it is hereby declared that nothing in this Act is to be taken to affect the law relating to murder or manslaughter or the operation of Section 2 of the Suicide Act 1961 (c. 60) (assisting suicide).

This would count against both active euthanasia (where the doctor or carer intentionally kills the person for that person's alleged benefit) and assisted suicide (where the doctor or carer provides the person with the information and means to take his own life with the intention that the information given will be used for this purpose).

There are two points to consider in the arguments put forward by those worried by the prospect of euthanasia. Both points shed light on aspects of the MCA to do with best interests. First, it is argued that best interests should be characterised more objectively. Instead of just talking of wishes and feelings or beliefs and values (see below), more overt reference should be made to protecting life, preserving health and preventing suffering, which are regarded as more objective aspects of best interests (SPUC, 2005). Secondly, the concern is that the Act might encourage the pendulum to swing in favour of hastening death 'by omission' (i.e. intentionally causing death by not providing necessary and customary treatment and care), especially where the person has stipulated that they do not wish to be kept alive, either by way of an advance refusal of treatment, or in an advance statement (see below), or via a LPA.

These two points are most squarely faced in Section 5.31 of the Code, which it is worth quoting at length.

Code of Practice, paragraph 5.31

All reasonable steps, which are in the person's best interests, should be taken to prolong their life. There will be a limited number of cases where treatment is futile, overly burdensome to the patient or where there is no prospect of recovery. In circumstances such as these, it may be that an assessment of best interests leads to the conclusion that it would be in the best interests of the patient to withdraw or withhold life-sustaining treatment, even if this may result in the person's death. The decision-maker must make a decision based on the best interests of the person who lacks capacity.

The first and last sentences of this passage reaffirm the intention expressed in Section 4(5). It has to be understood that when the Act talks of 'best interests', it does not refer to some single aspect that might contribute to a person's best interests, it rather refers to the outcome of the process of determination. In other words, it refers to everything involved in the checklist. Hence, the decision maker must not consider the person's age and appearance, but must consider 'all the relevant circumstances' and must not be motivated 'by a desire to bring about [the person's] death', and so on. This should go some way towards allaying fears that the Act is not explicitly interested in protecting life, preserving health and preventing suffering. Those who might be tempted to demand active euthanasia are thwarted by the clauses quoted from the Act above, specifically those prohibiting such action. The Code is overt about prolonging life, saying that 'all reasonable steps' should be taken, which argues in favour of protecting life. Similarly, if a person is suffering, it is hard not to conceive that this would be one of the 'relevant circumstances' that had to be considered. Furthermore, it seems unlikely that the alleviation of suffering would be something that the person him or herself (let alone a carer or relative) would oppose. Hence, it is difficult to imagine that the Act would in any sense encourage, when considering a person's best interests, that suffering be ignored. Therefore, there are a number of ways in which it is possible to argue that the MCA is distinctly on the side of protecting life, preserving health and preventing suffering.

It might still, however, be a concern that the Act could encourage euthanasia by omission. As has already been mentioned, a person may stipulate (through an LPA, an advance decision to refuse treatment, or by a statement of values) that he or she does not wish to be treated under certain circumstances. The real concern is that people should not be left to die, when they might otherwise survive. It is easy to imagine how this might occur in the face of very clear prior statements by the person, or by the donee of a LPA. And this, it is argued, might amount to euthanasia by omission, as it were, by the back door.

There are four points to note in response, all of which tell us something about the intentions of the MCA. First, as the passage from the Code quoted above (paragraph 5.31) makes plain, there will be a 'limited number' of cases where it is right to withdraw or withhold life-sustaining treatment, but this will only be if it is in the person's best interests. As we have seen, best interests have to be interpreted broadly by the application of the checklist, which includes the proviso that the determination of best interests should not 'be motivated by a desire to bring about [the person's] death'. In this sense, best interests cannot aim at the death of someone, even if the outcome of the decision is that the person dies. In essence, it can be argued, this makes use of the *doctrine of double effect*: the intention must always be to pursue the person's best interests, even if a foreseen consequence is that the person will die.

Furthermore, this makes the point, which is often repeated in medical ethics, that there is no real moral difference between doing and not doing something. In this case, whether you are doing something or whether you are withholding something, if you are 'motivated by a desire to bring about [the person's] death', you are breaking the law. The difference between intending something (implied by the idea of being 'motivated by a desire to bring about' something) and foreseeing it is sometimes regarded as *mere* semantics. But it makes the world of difference. One way to understand this is to consider that whether something is intended or only foreseen is not solely determined by what the person thinks at the time of doing or not doing whatever it is. The *nature* of the action itself is also important. A carefully titrated dose of analgesia to relieve pain is quite different from a large intravenous injection of potassium chloride putatively for the same purpose, whatever the doctor may claim he or she was thinking.

The starting point in any best interests determination regarding life-sustaining treatment is that there is a strong presumption that it is in the best interests of the person to stay alive.[6] The passage from the Code makes clear that withdrawing or withholding life-sustaining treatment would only be licit if it were 'futile, overly burdensome to the patient or where there is no prospect of recovery' (paragraph 5.31). The second point to note, therefore, is that this reflects another long-established doctrine of medical ethics, namely the *doctrine of ordinary and extraordinary means*. This states that we are bound to take ordinary means to help people, but there is no moral obligation to take extraordinary means. 'Extraordinary' implies a disproportion between the treatment and its likely outcome (which would include the treatment's being futile), or where the treatment (or investigation) was likely to be too burdensome for the patient. The MCA, therefore, reflects currently accepted and long-established doctrines of medical ethics concerning when life-sustaining treatments might be denied a person or stopped.[7]

The third point is that the MCA brings together in statute law much that was scattered in common law. For instance, it should not be forgotten that it has been the case for some while that a valid and applicable advance directive (or advance decision (AD) as it is now termed under the MCA) should be followed. In law, it is viewed in the same way as a contemporaneous refusal of treatment made by a competent adult. The best interests standard is therefore not relevant in these circumstances, as the creator of the AD has made his own competent best interests known before the onset of incapacity. However, even if the person's wishes at the end of life are not considered to be legally binding (remembering that ADs relating to life-sustaining treatment must comply with certain formalities under the MCA), the informal views of the person (the values statements described below) would, if known, still carry weight and might be an important factor to be weighed by a decision maker in any best interests decision to withdraw or withhold treatment (Code of Practice, paragraphs 5.32 and 5.34). In turn, this reflects the emphasis given to personal autonomy in medical ethics. If this is the decision the person would have made, and if we cherish personal decision-making, then we should honour it (whilst bearing in mind the caveats that should preclude assisted suicide, manslaughter or murder).

Any statements made by the person, therefore, or any written statements, should be given due weight and taken into account (Code of Practice, paragraphs 5.32 and 5.34). But the fourth point is that, in determining best interests, the doctor must always apply the checklist rather than reach an impression on the basis of a single piece of evidence.

> Doctors must apply the best interests' checklist and use their professional skills to decide whether life-sustaining treatment is in the person's best interests.
>
> (Code of Practice, paragraph 5.33)

And it might be that, in making a professional judgement or in applying the checklist, the doctor or other professionals involved do not feel that the decision being taken is what the person would have wanted, and not, overall, in his or her best interests. Contrariwise, others might feel that the doctor's decision is not in the person's best interests. In either case, the Act allows that the matter should be settled by the Court of Protection, but only as a last resort (Code, paragraph 5.33). Indeed, if anyone feels that the person's best interests are not being served, then there is a legal imperative that these doubts should be made plain and considered.

Case study 3.5 Withholding treatment in severe dementia

Mr Jordan has severe dementia and has been totally dependent for all his personal care for a number of years. He is immobile and doubly incontinent and is living in a continuing care unit where he had been placed some years before when his behaviour was often agitated and occasionally aggressive. He develops symptoms and signs suggestive of a chest infection. Although he has a mild fever, he continues to eat when fed and he is as alert as he has been for some months. His son and daughter have informed the consultant in charge of his care that he was never keen on seeing doctors and did not tend to take medications, even when prescribed, long before he became unwell with dementia. They also know, from things their father said when he was first diagnosed, that he would not wish to be kept alive unnecessarily.

Nevertheless, having reviewed his clinical state and discussed matters with the nurses and with the family, it is felt appropriate to prescribe oral antibiotics on the grounds that they will shorten the course of the chest infection, thereby reducing his suffering. It is not thought that he is likely to die from the infection. Having consulted with all concerned and reviewed all of the relevant circumstances, the decision to treat him is made in his best interests.

Five months later, having been a little less responsive for only about a day, Mr Jordan becomes acutely unwell. He rapidly becomes unresponsive, looks very toxic, is diagnosed as having developed pneumonia, probably caused by aspiration, and is soon comatose. Having gone through the checklist, on this occasion it is decided that oral antibiotics are unlikely to

Case study 3.5 (*cont.*)

be effective, whilst intravenous antibiotics (which would necessitate transfer to a medical ward in the nearby hospital) would be burdensome and might still not bring about a recovery. Hence, in his best interests, antibiotic treatment is withheld and palliative measures (tepid sponging and paracetamol) are taken. Mr Jordan dies after two days of illness.[8]

The person's views

The principles underpinning the MCA make it clear that the person who lacks capacity must be considered centre stage. In determining best interests, this is also apparent. 'So far as is reasonably ascertainable' whoever is deciding what might be in a person's best interests must consider:

- the person's past and present wishes and feelings (and, in particular, any relevant written statement made by him when he had capacity);
- the beliefs and values that would be likely to influence his decision if he had capacity; and
- the other factors that he would be likely to consider if he were able to do so (Section 4(6)).

One immediate point to note is the use again of the notion of ascertaining only what might be reasonable.

Case study 3.6 Haemorrhagic shock

A young female victim of a car crash is brought into casualty unconscious and with multiple traumas. There is a suspicion that she might be bleeding internally with evidence of increasing shock. She has no form of identification. Decisions to treat her have to be made immediately and it is not possible to delay in order to ascertain what her past wishes and feelings might have been, nor the beliefs and values that might have shaped her decisions about treatment.

As the Code makes clear,

> What is available in an emergency will be different to what is available in a non-emergency. But even in an emergency, there may still be an opportunity to try to communicate with the person or his friends or carers.
>
> (Code of Practice, paragraph 5.39)

The Code goes on to say that the person's views might be demonstrated by their behaviour; certainly, undue influence should not distort the person's views (paragraph 5.40). Views can be made known, not only by verbal accounts, but also perhaps by audio recordings (paragraph 5.41). But there is a special emphasis on written records.

Written statements do not need to take a particular form, unless they are advance refusals of life-sustaining treatment (MCA, Section 25(5–6)). The importance of the clause in Section 4(6) about relevant written statements is that this brings into consideration all advance statements, not just refusals of treatment. Hence, the potential importance of what are often called 'values statements'.[9] In such a statement, a person might record any values or beliefs that could help someone at a later date to decide on what the person would want even though he/she could not participate in decision-making. As is well known, although people can *refuse* treatment, and under the MCA, they can do this in advance of the situation arising, no one has the right to *demand* specific treatment. However, in a statement of values, a person is at liberty to express any views at all, including the view that he or she might wish treatment to be pursued for as long as possible under all circumstances.

A real example of some relevance here is that of Mr Leslie Burke, who challenged the General Medical Council over its guidance on withdrawing and withholding treatment (GMC, 2002). Mr Burke suffered from motor neurone disease and was concerned that he might find himself in a situation where he could not communicate, but where a feeding tube was being withdrawn against his wishes. Mr Burke lost his case on appeal (*Mr Leslie Burke v. GMC*).[10] Section 4(6) of the MCA, which stipulates that the person determining best interests 'must consider ... in particular, any relevant written statement', would have allowed Mr Burke to express his concerns and would have ensured that they were given a good deal of weight. In the light of the case, and to take account of the MCA, the GMC updated its guidance in its document *Treatment and Care towards the End of Life* (GMC, 2010).

Nevertheless, any such advance statement would have to be seen in context, and it remains the case that the broader notion of best interests implies that those making decisions for someone who lacks capacity should take into account all of the factors that might arise from following the checklist. Therefore, under certain circumstances, doctors might not have to follow a written request, although they may have to justify and record their reasons for not doing so (Code of Practice, paragraph 5.43).

> they would not have to follow a written request if they think the specific treatment would be clinically unnecessary or not appropriate for the person's condition, so not in the person's best interests.
>
> (Code of Practice, paragraph 5.44)

As previously discussed, a person's wishes, feelings, beliefs and values when known, should always to be afforded great respect. A post legislative review of the MCA carried out by the House of Lords Select Committee in 2014 concluded that a general lack of awareness of the provision of Section 4(6) has meant that the views of the person are not always considered in practice:

> Best interests decision-making is often not undertaken in the way set out in the Act: the wishes, thoughts and feelings of [the incapacitated person] are not routinely prioritised. Instead, clinical judgements or resource-led decision-making predominate. The least restrictive option is not routinely or adequately considered.
>
> (House of Lords 2014, Conclusions and Recommendations, page 8, paragraph 3)

Justice Peter Jackson summarised the importance of a person's wishes and feelings in the case of *Wye Valley NHS Trust* v. *Mrs B* in 2015,

> As the Act and the European Convention make clear, a conclusion that a person lacks decision-making capacity is not an 'off-switch' for his rights and freedoms. To state the obvious, the wishes and feelings, beliefs and values of people with mental disability are as important to them as they are to anyone else, and may even be more important. It would therefore be wrong in principle to apply any automatic discount to their point of view.

The Code goes on to note that 'Everybody's values and beliefs influence the decisions they make' and it suggests (paragraph 5.46) that evidence of someone's beliefs and values might be found in their:

- cultural background
- religious beliefs
- political convictions or
- past behaviour or habits.

Case study 3.7   Jasmine's depression

Jasmine has a history of recurrent depression. She always attends outpatients with a member of her family and when she has capacity; she has made it plain that she values family support. The closeness of the family is in keeping with cultural norms for someone of Jasmine's background. On this occasion, she is admitted to hospital with a severe depression. She has become almost mute, refusing to talk to anyone. When it comes to a multidisciplinary meeting, which Jasmine is invited to attend on the ward, her cousin (who has previously come to outpatients with her) wishes to accompany her. But, although she indicates no objections, Jasmine's consent to her cousin taking part is not forthcoming because she will not readily communicate. Given that she is unable to communicate a decision, it is deemed that she lacks capacity in this regard and a judgement about best interests has to be made. The team do not feel that anything will be discussed that it might be prejudicial for Jasmine's cousin to hear, they feel it might be supportive for Jasmine herself and, on the basis of their previous knowledge of Jasmine's feelings about being accompanied and of the cultural appropriateness of such support for Jasmine, it is judged in her best interests for her cousin to accompany her during the meeting.

Section 4(6)(c) of the MCA requires decision makers to consider 'other factors' the person might have considered if able. According to the Code,

> This might include the effect of the decision on other people, obligations to dependants or the duties of a responsible citizen.
>
> (Code of Practice, paragraph 5.47)

Therefore, it is permissible to consider actions that might benefit others,

> *as long as they are in the best interests of the person who lacks* capacity to make the decision . . . 'Best interests' goes beyond the person's medical interests.
>
> (Code of Practice, paragraph 5.48)

Case study 3.8   Early onset dementia and genetic testing

A man develops dementia at the age of 46. Four years later, a new genetic marker for some early onset dementias is discovered, but the man does not have the capacity to give consent for a blood test to be taken for the purpose of testing him. However, his family are keen to know whether he carries the genetic trait. It might be considered in his best interests to perform the test because it is reasonable to assume that the interests of his dependants would be a factor he would consider if able.

The Code records that courts have previously ruled that wider benefits might include,

providing or gaining emotional support from a close relationship.

(Code of Practice, paragraph 5.48)

Case study 3.9 Down's syndrome and the day centre

A young woman, Jill, with Down's syndrome has been attending a particular day centre for a couple of years and has built up a friendship with another woman who attends the centre. However, the friend moves house and starts to attend an alternative day centre, which she can be taken to more easily by her relatives. Jill is noticeably dejected. For Jill to attend the alternative day centre to be with her friend, she will need to pay for the extra transport. She lacks the capacity to make decisions about her finances, but it is decided on her behalf that, since she would clearly benefit from the emotional support of being with her friend, it is in her best interests to use her money to get her to the new day centre.

Consulting others

The MCA is quite specific about the people who must be consulted, 'if it is practicable and appropriate', about what might be in the person's best interests. In particular, people should be consulted about the matters mentioned in Section 4(6), which concern the person's past and present wishes and feelings, beliefs and values and other relevant factors (as discussed above).

MCA, Section 4(7)

The views of the following must be taken into account:

(a) anyone named by the person as someone to be consulted on the matter in question or on matters of that kind,
(b) anyone engaged in caring for the person or interested in his welfare,
(c) any donee of a lasting power of attorney granted by the person, and
(d) any deputy appointed for the person by the court.

We are reminded in the Code of Practice that if there is no one to speak about the person's best interests, in some circumstances – where serious medical decisions are being made or decisions that might lead to a change in the person's place of residence – the person may require an independent mental capacity advocate (IMCA) to be appointed. The Code goes on to make a number of points about good practice:

- 'decision-makers must show they have thought carefully about who to speak to' (paragraph 5.51);
- decision-makers should have a clear record of their reasons for not speaking to a particular person if they fall within the list given in Section 4(7) of the Act (paragraph 5.51);
- careful consideration should be given to the views of family carers (paragraph 5.51);
- at the end of the process, decision-makers should record why they thought the specific decision was in the person's best interests, especially if the decision goes against the views of someone consulted (paragraph 5.52).

The Code suggests, in paragraph 5.53, two aspects that the decision maker should be enquiring about:

- 'what the people consulted think is in the person's best interests in this matter, and
- if they can give information on the person's wishes and feelings, beliefs and values.'

The significance of this is that it suggests the Act is concerned about both objective factors and substituted judgements (see above). The decision maker is to enquire about what someone 'thinks is in the person's best interests', which is distinct from enquiring what they think the person him/herself would have thought. In other words, although the views of the person concerned who lacks capacity are vitally important, the decision maker needs to be open to the views of others too.

Case study 3.10 Agitation and aggression

Mr Hodgson developed dementia six years ago. He continues to live with his wife who, like him, is aged 78 years. Over the last few months, towards evening, he has become irritable and aggressive. Mr Hodgson's sister-in-law calls every day and is very concerned about her sister. She thinks Mr Hodgson should be in long-term care. Mrs Hodgson is keen, however, to keep her husband at home for as long as possible.

Having had no success with alternative psychosocial strategies, the consultant agrees to try psychotropic medication, having explained the possible side effects. The response is monitored by the community psychiatric nurse (CPN), who has been involved for a long while. Mr Hodgson does indeed show evidence of some side effects after only a few weeks. Although the irritability and obvious aggression have lessened, he is somewhat sedated and slightly unsteady.

In making a decision about whether or not to continue with the medication, the consultant talks with the CPN, who feels the situation is less volatile and the side effects not so severe as to warrant the drug being stopped. The sister-in-law still feels that things are getting too much for her sister and she wishes Mr Hodgson was in a home. When the consultant talks with Mrs Hodgson, she reiterates her desire to keep her husband at home for as long as possible, she is not very concerned about the side effects and she recalls Mr Hodgson himself saying how he would hate being put in a home. Overall, the consultant also feels the medication is the best option, and, given everyone's views, it is decided that this is in Mr Hodgson's best interests. The reason for not accepting the sister-in-law's view is noted: not only does it not reflect the previous wishes and feelings of Mr Hodgson, nor the current views of Mrs Hodgson, but also keeping him at home, albeit slightly sedated in the evenings, is the least restrictive option and therefore in keeping with one of the principles of the MCA.

There are two further points of importance to be noted. First, whilst it is clear that attorneys appointed under a LPA or an Enduring Power of Attorney (EPA), or a deputy appointed by a court must make the decision in connection with the matter they have been appointed to deal with, if practicable and appropriate, they should also be consulted on other issues. They might, for instance, be able to shed light on the person's previous wishes, beliefs, values and feelings or the existence of an advance decision refusing treatment, for example. Secondly, although the thrust of the MCA is that there should be broad consultation in order to determine the person's best interests, professionals must still abide by codes of practice or guidelines concerning confidentiality. Only those with 'a proper interest in having the information in question'[11] should be consulted and they only need to be informed about confidential matters insofar as it is necessary. The best interests of the person without capacity remain central.

At several points already in this chapter, the issue of the views of the family have emerged as important. There is, of course, a relationship between the individual's best interests and the best interests of his or her family. But this relationship is not always straightforward. There might, for instance, be disagreements within a family. Even setting aside the worry that some section of the family might be motivated by malign intent, self-interest may well exist in the most benign atmosphere. If a parent goes into long-term care, for instance, there may be a complex mixture of emotional, financial and social consequences for the family: less to inherit, further to travel for one daughter but less far for another, fewer disturbances at night, resentment expressed by the mother towards her daughter (for not taking her in to live), but not towards her son, and so on. Interests collide and need to be negotiated around the person concerned who should remain centre stage (Emmett *et al.*, 2014).

There is a deeper sense, however, in which the best interests of the person and his or her family routinely overlap:

> interests are often complex and intertwined. In a family, it will rarely be the case that a single person's interests always take priority: rather some consideration will be given to everyone's interests and some degree of compromise found. The Mental Capacity Act reflects this reality in its broad approach to 'best interests'. A determination of a person's best interests is not limited simply to what, in the abstract, might seem best for their personal welfare or well-being, but also includes consideration of factors such as their beliefs and values ... and other factors they might have taken into account themselves. In many cases, this will include strong concern for the welfare of others in their family ... [T]here can be no legal or ethical duty to continue caring where this is no longer physically or emotionally viable.
>
> (Nuffield Council on Bioethics, 2009, paragraphs 7.35–7.37)

On this basis, the Nuffield Council's report recommended that professionals should play a role in supporting family carers to consider their own needs.

The philosophical basis for this is the notion of 'relational autonomy'. It is, after all, the notion of 'autonomy' (i.e. self-rule) that places the person centre stage. But, strictly speaking, none of us is entirely autonomous; our autonomy is 'relational'. For we are always situated in a culture, history, geography, social group, legal system and so forth (Hughes, 2001). And we are typically situated in a family, so there is an inevitable sense in which best interests overlap. In a study of family carers of people with dementia, one wife said of her husband 'My best interests ... are his best interests' (Hughes *et al.*, 2002). Best interests, therefore, do not always collide, they often coincide. Thus, to understand the person's best interests will frequently require an understanding of the family's social and cultural background.

Restricting rights and acting reasonably

Deciding what is best for a person who lacks capacity can seem like a daunting task. In some ways, this is how it should be and hence it is important that the checklist is followed. However, Section 4(9) of the Act establishes that the decision maker will act within the law if he or she 'reasonably believes' that the decision or action 'is in the best interests of the person concerned'.

In fact, in the next Section (5), entitled 'Acts in connection with care or treatment', it sets out that if 'reasonable steps' have been taken to establish that the person lacks capacity and if someone giving care or treatment 'reasonably believes' that the person lacks capacity and that the care or treatment is in the person's best interests, then it would be as if the person him/herself had consented to the treatment. In other words, Section 5 of the MCA provides the carer or clinician with protection from liability insofar as the steps taken and the beliefs about the person's capacity and best interests are reasonable.

Continuing the theme of reasonableness, Section 6 of the MCA allows that a person can be restrained under two circumstances:

- if there is a reasonable belief that it is necessary to restrain the person to prevent him or her from coming to harm;
- if the act of restraint is proportionate to the likelihood of harm and to the seriousness of that harm.

Thus, it might be entirely reasonable to ensure that doors are locked in a home where it would be unsafe for people to get outside. Nevertheless, even if this section allows restraint in the sense of restrictions of liberty, it does not allow deprivation of liberty – a topic to which we shall return in Chapter 4.

Making the best interests judgement

Making decisions about a person's best interests might be very straightforward, but the decisions can be enormously difficult too, either because of the complexity of the task (e.g. if there are complicated financial matters to be dealt with), or because of disagreement amongst those concerned. Given the number of decisions that might have to be made for someone because of lack of capacity can be vast, there may have to be numerous decision makers. The *Code* suggests various different types of decision-making (paragraph 5.8):

- day-to-day decisions by 'the carer most directly involved with the person at the time';
- medical decisions by doctors and other healthcare staff;
- nursing decisions or decisions by paid carers;
- decisions by attorneys (under a LPA or EPA) or deputies appointed by a court.

It also suggests that there will be times when 'a joint decision might be made by a number of people' (paragraph 5.11). If there are disputes, it will be up to the decision maker to try to reach some form of consensus, not by disregarding anyone's concerns, but by balancing them (paragraph 6.64). There are various ways in which a decision maker's conclusion might be challenged. Paragraph 5.68 of the Code sets out the options:

- an advocate might be involved;
- a second opinion sought;
- a formal or informal 'best interests' case conference could be held;
- there could be some form of mediation;
- formal complaint procedures might be used;
- the matter might be referred to the Court of Protection as a last resort.

In the main, however, it will be up to the decision maker, who must act in the person's best interests. And the normal way to ensure that this is arrived at in a suitably inclusive and broad way is to follow the steps outlined by the checklist. Figure 3.1 depicts the checklist, and what it entails, as a flow diagram. Not every step would be possible or appropriate in every case, but (as we have seen) *reasonable* steps must be taken before it can *reasonably* be said that the decision is in a person's best interests.

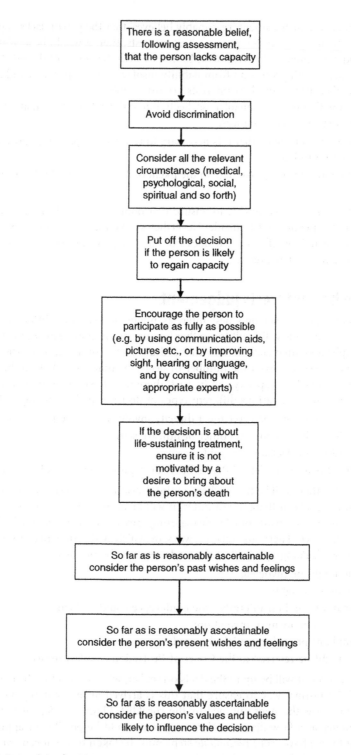

Figure 3.1 Determining best interests

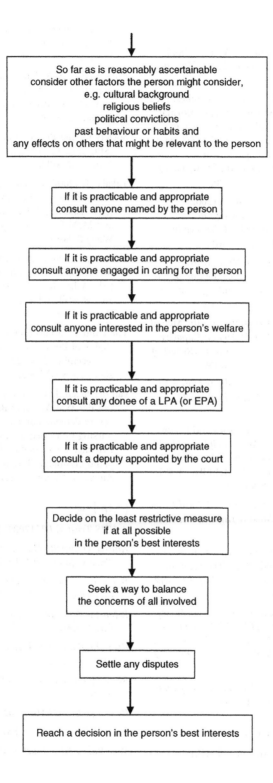

Figure 3.1 *(cont.)*

References

Department of Constitutional Affairs (2007) Mental Capacity Act 2005, Code of Practice, London: HMSO.

Emmett, C., Poole, M., Bond, J. & Hughes, J. C. (2014) A Relative Safeguard? The informal roles that families and carers play when patients with dementia are discharged from hospital into care in England and Wales. *International Journal of Law, Policy and the Family*, 28(3), 302–320.

General Medical Council (GMC) (2002) *Withholding and Withdrawing Life-Prolonging Treatments: Good Practice in Decision-Making*. London: GMC.

General Medical Council (GMC) (2010) *Treatment and Care Towards the End of Life: Good Practice in Decision Making*. London: GMC. www.gmc-uk.org/index.asp.

House of Lords Select Committee on the Mental Capacity Act 2005 (2014) *Mental Capacity Act 2005: Post-Legislative Scrutiny (Report of Session 2013-14)*. London: HMSO.

Hughes, J. C. (2001) Views of the person with dementia. *Journal of Medical Ethics*, 27, 86–91.

Hughes, J. C. (2007) Ethical issues and health care for older people. In: *Principles of Health Care Ethics* (2nd edn.) (eds. Ashcroft, R. E., Dawson, A., Draper, H. & McMillan, J. R.), pp. 469–474. John Wiley & Sons.

Hughes, J. C. & Baldwin, C. (2006) *Ethical Issues in Dementia Care: Making Difficult Decisions*. Jessica Kingsley.

Hughes, J. C., Hope, T., Reader, S. & Rice, D. (2002) Dementia and ethics: The views of informal carers. *Journal of the Royal Society of Medicine*, 95, 242–246.

John, S. D. (2007) Ordinary and extraordinary means. In: *Principles of Health Care Ethics* (2nd edn.) (eds. Ashcroft, R. E., Dawson, A., Draper, H. and McMillan, J. R.), pp. 269–272. John Wiley & Sons.

Law Commission (2017) *Mental Capacity and Deprivation of Liberty* (Law Com 372), London: HMSO.

Mental Capacity Act 2005, c.9.

Mental Capacity Amendment Bill [HL] 2017–19.

Nuffield Council on Bioethics (2009) *Dementia: Ethical Issues*. London: Nuffield Council on Bioethics.

Ruck-Keene, A. & Auckland, C. (2015) More presumptions please? Wishes, feelings and best interests decision-making. *Elder Law Journal*, 293–301.

Society for the Protection of the Unborn Child (SPUC) (2005) *The Mental Capacity Act 2005 Explained*. SPUC.

Takala, T. (2007) Acts and omissions. In: *Principles of Health Care Ethics* (2nd edn.) (eds. Ashcroft, R. E., Dawson, A., Draper, H. and McMillan, J. R.), pp. 273–276. John Wiley & Sons.

Uniacke, S. (2007) The doctrine of double effect. In: *Principles of Health Care Ethics* (2nd edn.) (eds. Ashcroft, R. E., Dawson, A., Draper, H. and McMillan, J. R.), pp. 263–268. John Wiley & Sons.

The United Nations (2006) Convention on the Rights of Persons with Disabilities (adopted 13 December 2006, entered into force 3 May 2008) 2515 UNTS 3.

van der Steen, J. T., Ooms, M. E., Mehr, D. R., van der Wal, W. G. & Ribbe, M. W. (2002) Severe dementia and adverse outcomes of nursing home-acquired pneumonia: Evidence for mediation by functional and pathophysiological decline. *Journal of the American Geriatrics Society*, 50, 439–448.

Case law

A NHS Trust v. *DU* [2009] EWHC 3504 (Fam).

Aintree University Hospitals NHS Foundation Trust v. *James* [2013] UKSC 67.

Burke, R (on the application of) v. *General Medical Council & Ors* [2005] EWCA Civ 1003.

R (on the Application of Stevens) v. *Plymouth City Council & Anor* [2002] EWCA Civ 388.

RB v. *Brighton and Hove City Council* [2014] EWCA Civ 561.

Re AK (Gift Application) [2014] EWHC B11 (COP).

Re GC [2008] EWHC 3402 (Fam).

Re M; ITW v. *Z* [2009] EWHC 2525 (Fam).

Wye Valley NHS Trust v. *Mr B* [2015] EWCOP 60.

Notes

1 Lord Justice Jackson described Section 1(6) as a necessary 'brake on excessive use of the powers vested in local authorities and the court' in *RB* v. *Brighton and Hove City Council* [2014] EWCA Civ 561 at para. 51.

2 See *Aintree* v. *James* [2013] UKSC 67 at para. 39.

3 See *Re M; ITW* v. *Z* [2009] EWHC 2525 (Fam) at para. 32.

4 See *A NHS Trust* v. *DU* [2009] EWHC 3504 (Fam) at para. 10.

5 *See Re GC* [2008] EWHC 3402 (Fam) (Hedley J) at para. 21.

6 See *Aintree* v. *James* at para. 41

7 This is not to deny, however, that there are arguments about these doctrines themselves, as might be expected (John, 2007; Takala, 2007; Uniacke, 2007); nor is it to claim that the decisions that have to be made will be straightforward (for further discussion in the context of dementia and older people see Hughes & Baldwin, 2006; and Hughes, 2007). It is appropriate that there is intellectual debate about principles and doctrines and inevitable that, in a field of complex and conflicting values, working out the appropriate action or decision should not be glibly undertaken. Nevertheless, it cannot be said that the MCA ushers in a disregard of basic ethical doctrines or principles. Indeed, somewhat to the contrary, it can be argued that the MCA ushers in a much-needed recognition of the human rights of those who find it difficult to make decisions for themselves for whatever reason.

8 There is, indeed, evidence that clinicians do make fine distinctions concerning whether antibiotics should be withheld, used palliatively, or used with curative intent in cases of pneumonia in dementia (van der Steen *et al.*, 2002).

9 Various values statements exist and can be found on the Internet. In the UK, the Department of Health's website contains the End of Life Strategy which highlights the usefulness of the 'Preferred Priorities of Care' document.

10 The Court of Appeal made it plain that doctors are under no legal obligation to provide treatment at the patient's request if the treatment is not thought to be in the patient's best interests.

11 *R (on the application of Stevens)* v. *Plymouth City Council & Anor* [2002] EWCA Civ 388 at para. 49.

Deprivation of Liberty Safeguards: Past, Present and Future

Susan F. Welsh

Introduction

The Deprivation of Liberty Safeguards (DoLS) are a legal framework that exists to ensure that individuals who lack the requisite capacity to consent to the arrangements for their care, where such care may (because of restrictions imposed on an individual's freedom of choice or movement) amount to a 'deprivation of liberty', have the arrangements independently assessed to ensure they are in the best interests of the individual concerned. (Mental Capacity Act (MCA) 2005: Deprivation of Liberty Safeguards (England) Annual report 2014–2015 Health and Social care information centre)

The DoLS framework is contained in Schedule 1A to the Mental Capacity Act (MCA) 2005 and applies to all hospitals (general and psychiatric) and care homes (including private care homes) but not to deprivation of liberty in supported living, shared lives, and private and domestic settings. The hospital and care home must apply for authorisation of deprivation of liberty from the 'supervisory body' (local authorities in England and in Wales but to the Local Health Board for hospital deprivation of liberty in Wales).

The 'Bournewood Gap'

Since a learning disabled man, admitted to Bournewood Hospital in Surrey (*HL* v. *UK*), successfully challenged his 'informal' 'detention' in a psychiatric hospital, citing his right to liberty and security of person under Section 5(1) of the Human Rights Act (HRA) 1998, and his right to challenge his confinement, under Section 5(4), both of which were breached, the Deprivation of Liberty Safeguards (DoLS) has taken on a life of its own.

The *HL* case identified a group of people who lacked capacity to consent to treatment and who were being deprived of their liberty for the purpose of providing treatment for their mental disorder under the common law and not under the Mental Health Act (MHA) 1983. This group was being denied the procedural safeguards demanded by Article 5 of the European Convention on Human Rights (ECHR). As a qualified right (as opposed to absolute), Article 5 permits detention of persons of 'unsound mind' but this must be in accordance with a procedure prescribed by law. The ECHR was incorporated into UK law in the Human Rights Act (HRA) 1998 (that came into force in 2000).

The key finding in the case of *HL* was that a lack of objection to deprivation of liberty should not be regarded as equivalent to consent (*HL* v. *UK*). In order to guarantee that a deprivation of liberty is not arbitrary, it must be undertaken in a manner that is prescribed by national law, and compliant with the provisions of the ECHR.

MCA amendments and development of Deprivation of Liberty Safeguards: the past

The subsequent amendment to the Mental Capacity Act (MCA) (to ensure future compliance of all state authorities with ECHR) was achieved in Schedule 1A, inserted by the vehicle of the Mental Health Act 2007 and comprising 13 parts; an administrative procedure that provides legal authority for a deprivation of liberty. A separate Code of Practice accompanied it. The Deprivation of Liberty Safeguards was born and the early years are detailed in the former edition of this book.

As a basic refresher, to require the authorisation that the DoLS provides, the person must be aged 18 or over, and the first condition is that a person ('P') is detained in a hospital or care home for the purpose of being given care or treatment, in circumstances which amount to deprivation of the person's liberty.[1]

Unsound mind is taken, in DoLS, to mean 'mental disorder' in accordance with the definition of *mental disorder* in the MHA 1983. This was changed by the MHA 2007 (as of 3 November 2008) so that it is no longer split into the four classifications of mental illness, psychopathic disorder, mental impairment and severe mental impairment. Section 1 now states that: 'mental disorder' means any disorder or disability of the mind. There are, however, two exceptions. Abnormally aggressive or seriously irresponsible conduct is a consideration for learning disability (not personality disorder). Learning disability is therefore not a 'mental disorder' unless associated with this conduct. Some exclusions to definition of mental disorder have been removed but dependence on alcohol or drugs is still excluded from the category of 'mental disorder'.[2]

Deprivation or restriction?

In *Guzzardi* v. *Italy*, the European Court of Human Rights (ECtHR) in Strasbourg held that, in determining whether situations constituted a deprivation of liberty, regard must be had for a 'whole range of criteria such as the type, duration, effects and manner of implementation of the (restrictive) measure in question'. The court in *Guzzardi* asserted that the distinction between restriction on liberty and deprivation of liberty was 'merely one of degree or intensity, and not one of nature or substance'.

The Code of Practice[3] accompanying the Deprivation of Liberty Safeguards legislation provides examples of acts that may, *when taken together*, under principles as above, amount to a deprivation of liberty, including;

1. The person is not allowed to leave the hospital or care home. Restrictions that are put in place for the person's protection would not necessarily amount to a deprivation of liberty.
2. The person has no or very limited choice about their life within the care home or hospital staff exercise control over assessments, treatment, care and movement within the environment.
3. The person is not able to maintain contact with the world outside of hospital or care home staff exercise control over contacts/access to other people.
4. Restraint is/was used on admission and the person is not realistically allowed to leave. Carers would not be allowed to discharge.

(This must be read in conjunction with recent case law specifying the 'acid test' that constitutes deprivation of liberty, and which will be discussed more fully later in this chapter (Supreme Court *Cheshire West and Chester Council* v. *P*).

Additionally, the Code of Practice specifies that the duration of restrictions is of paramount importance in deciding whether they constitute deprivation of liberty; actions that are immediately necessary to prevent harm may not, in isolation, be sufficiently restrictive to constitute a deprivation of liberty. A prolonged journey to an institution or a period of travel that requires a person to be 'more than persuaded or restrained' (being neither too prolonged a restraint to justify a DoLS, nor too great a restriction to be lawful under MCA legislation) may, however, require a one-off order from the Court of Protection. The less autonomous an individual becomes within a care environment, the more that person moves towards a position of being deprived of their liberty.

Storck v. *Germany* defined three components of deprivation of liberty:

(a) The objective component of confinement in a particular restricted place for a not negligible length of time;
(b) The subjective component of lack of valid consent; and
(c) The attribution of responsibility to the state.

How not to deprive a person of their liberty

To avoid depriving persons of their liberty requires promotion of the following:

1. Maximisation of liberty and autonomy
2. Person-centred care
3. Involvement of family and friends
4. Minimising restrictions
5. Reviewing the care plan frequently

(also to be read in conjunction with the more up to date Supreme Court case law in *Cheshire West and Chester Council* v. *P*).

The mental health assessment at present must be done by a doctor, based on the case law of the European Court, which states that 'it must be convincingly shown on the basis of *objective medical expertise* that the person to be detained is mentally disordered' (*Wintwerp* v. *Netherlands*) in keeping with Article 5 that the deprivation of liberty may be permitted in persons of '*unsound mind*' according to law (i.e., within the framework of DoLS). Currently, the Mental Health Assessor must be Section 12(2) MHA-approved or a registered medical practitioner with three years of special experience of mental disorder diagnosis and treatment. In addition, the mental health assessor must have completed an approved (by the Secretary of State) mental health assessor training course.

Deprivation of Liberty Safeguards: the present

The *substance* of what does (and what does not) constitute a deprivation of liberty has evolved through case law since its inception in UK law, from its first constituent elements in the early days post *HL*, to the 2014 landmark decision of what is commonly known as the 'Cheshire West' case (*Cheshire West and Chester Council* v. *P*) that drew a line in the sand. Lady Hale determined that 'what it means to be deprived of liberty must mean the same for everyone . . . a gilded cage is still a cage' and in doing so, she and the Supreme Court vastly broadened the criteria for what constitutes a deprivation of liberty, as in what environments and in which ways care is delivered.

The acid test

The Supreme Court judgment in *Cheshire West* clarified the 'acid test' for what constitutes a deprivation of liberty. Where lack of capacity to consent to arrangements for care and treatment, continuous supervision and control and a lack of freedom to leave are all present together, the test is met.

Notably, in reference to the lower court judgments, irrelevant are compliance or lack of objection, the relative normality of the placements (whatever the comparison made), and the reason or purpose behind a particular placement.

Also (significantly), it held that a person can be deprived of his/her liberty in community (including shared living) and domestic settings (e.g. 24 hour care in a person's home that they lack capacity to consent to) when the State is responsible for such care arrangements. Such deprivations of liberty must be authorised by the Court of Protection. The acid test applies to patients in acute non-psychiatric hospitals too (*NHS Trust and others* v. *FG*). This judgment marked a significant change to previous established practice; however, of interest, the ECtHR has focused on deprivation of liberty for those with mental health problems in psychiatric hospitals and care homes only, and has not at any time given consideration to individuals being cared for in general hospitals, supported living, shared lives and private and domestic settings – this is unique to our own domestic courts.

Despite the challenges presented by *Cheshire West*, legally and ethically, DoLS seeks to ensure that those deprived of liberty are treated in a lawful way, and it provides a legal framework through which the decision to deprive anyone of their liberty can be challenged, compliant with ECHR.

The resultant fallout (experienced by local authorities particularly) has been substantial.

DoLS applications have risen steeply in England since *Cheshire West*. Overall, 195,840 DoLS applications were reported as having been received by Councils from 1 April 2015 to 31 March 2016. This is the most since the DoLS were introduced in 2009 and represent 454 DoLS applications received per 100,000 adults in England. In the previous year, the figure was 137,541, and prior to the 2014 Supreme Court judgment where the total number of applications received was 13,715 (Mental Capacity Act 2005).[4]

The practical resource implications of having enough assessors and being able to process applications within the required legal time frames have been considerable, notwithstanding the increased costs associated with the broadening of the criteria. In the East of England, for example, in 2015–2016 only 22% of applications were completed within the 21 days required and only 7% within the first seven days. Percentages of completed authorisations were 50% within three months, 29% in three to six months and 21% taking more than six months during that time period.[5]

Developments in case law have resulted in substantial financial burdens within the health and social care sector. In *Liverpool City Council, Nottinghamshire County Council, LB of Richmond upon Thames and Shropshire Council* v. *SSH*, local authorities sought a mandatory order, by means of judicial review, to require the Secretary of State for Health (SSH) to pay the annual shortfall, estimated to be between one third of a billion pounds and two thirds of a billion pounds for councils across the country as a result of *Cheshire West*. The action failed due to the delay in submitting the application, but it seems likely that with annual financial constraints already imposed upon local authorities by the State (before the extra costs of *Cheshire West*), they will be compelled to re-apply at a future date (within the necessary time frame).

Not only has *Cheshire West* broadened criteria for those individuals cared for in what previously was presumed to be less restrictive circumstances than would trigger a DoLS application, but case law has also evolved in parallel, and increasingly recognises where the application of DoLS is required in environments not previously even considered.

For example, considerable disquiet was expressed (Crews *et al.*, 2014) when it was confirmed that it is possible to deprive a person of their liberty in an intensive care setting, in relation to patients who were being cared for in circumstances that fulfilled the criteria. However, the Department of Health (DOH) (Department of Health Guidance, 2015) confirmed that DoLS can only be used where the individual has a mental disorder within the meaning of the MHA. A state of unconsciousness is not considered as a mental disorder for the purposes of schedule 1A, that is a person under anaesthetic who does not have a mental disorder is ineligible for DoLS. The DOH also confirmed that if a person reaching the last few weeks of their life gives capacitous consent to the arrangements for their care and treatment earlier in their treatment, this is taken to apply when they later lose capacity, hence DoLS does not apply (presuming there is no change to the care arrangements in place) (Department of Health Guidance, 2015).

When Maria Ferreira (who had a learning disability) died in an intensive care unit (ICU), her sister argued that a jury was required for the subsequent inquest because she was deprived of her liberty at the time of her death, which was a form of 'state detention' under Sections 7 and 48 of the Coroners and Justice Act (CJA) 2009. Whether 'state detention' equated to 'deprivation of liberty' under Article 5(1) ECHR was at issue, as was the relevance of *Cheshire West* to those particular circumstances.

Ms Ferreira was not in state detention according to the Court of Appeal for three alternative reasons: first, that *Cheshire West* did not apply; second, that if it did apply, she was free to leave; and, final, unlike MCA, Section 64(5) (references to deprivation of a person's liberty have the same meaning as in Article 5(1) of the Human Rights Convention), the CJA 2009 did not require consideration of Article 5 HRA 1998 and an intensive care unit (ICU) is not state detention. Moreover, *R (Ferreira)* v. *HM Senior Coroner for Inner South London* and others confirmed that a deprivation of liberty did not constitute state detention, an important distinction for families of those affected by the ruling.

Referring to *Winterwerp*, at issue is whether the unsoundness of mind justifies 'compulsory confinement' under Article 5(1) – in this case, it was argued that it was her physical illness that prevented her from leaving. The Court of Appeal held therefore that the acid test did not apply when the deprivation of liberty is on the basis of physical disorder rather than restrictions imposed by the hospital.

The case was in contrast to *NHS Trust I* v. *G* where a woman of 'unsound mind' was prevented from leaving a hospital and would be compelled (as necessary) to undergo a caesarean section. In that case, the circumstances amounted to a deprivation of liberty and authorisation was required, because the treatment was materially different from that given to a woman of 'sound mind'.

Since *Ferreira*, the law has been changed, brought about by the Policing and Crime Act 2017 (and the resultant subsequent amendment to Section 48 of Coroners and Justice Act (CJA) 2009). Previously, those individuals who died while subject to deprivation of their liberty were considered (by law) to be in 'state detention', which required a jury inquest. In 2015 alone, this led to an additional 7,183 inquests (Report of the Chief Coroner to the Lord Chancellor 2015–2016). By law, no routine inquests are now required, saving distress for families, and extra costs that have not benefitted the individual concerned. Paper inquests and discretion regarding post-mortems are applied in selected cases.

However, the Department of Health is set to introduce reforms to death certification in England and Wales. The announcement from England's Department of Health and Social Care on 11 June 2018 is that new local 'medical examiners' will from April 2019 start checking all death certificates for accuracy. This will introduce a form of scrutiny over all deaths that are not investigated by the coroner. It will require, among other processes, that death certificates are to be submitted in draft to those examiners and if it is their opinion that the death was attributable to failure of care (among other causes), then a referral to the coroner is made.[6] This would prevent any deaths of persons subject to deprivation of liberty (that could be due to poor care) from going unnoticed.

Since *Ferreira*, areas of healthcare that provide palliative care, and those which provide for disorders of consciousness, are not in fact depriving those individuals of their liberty, based on the conclusion that the patient is receiving the same physical health treatment as a person of 'sound mind', and, as has been stated previously, a state of unconsciousness does not constitute a mental disorder for the purposes of Schedule 1A MCA.

How to know when a person is (or is not) within scope of Article 5 HRA remains problematic however. For example, what constitutes 'unsound mind' and 'mental disorder' is not spelt out in case law judgments, especially given the judgment in *Briggs* v. *Briggs*, where, although viewed by the court as deprived of his liberty, did Paul Briggs suffer from 'mental disorder' or 'mental incapacity'? As someone receiving medical treatment for the after-effects of a motorcycle crash, he was arguably not deprived of his liberty – it was his physical condition that prevented him from leaving.

The eligibility criteria for DoLS as set out in paragraph 4.4[7] in Schedule 1A MCA has also presented its own challenges as it includes that 'a person is ineligible for DoLS if ... [he is] within the scope of the MHA and objecting to the proposed psychiatric treatment', with the DoLS assessor required to determine whether the proposed DoLS would authorise the person to be a 'mental health patient', that is a person accommodated in a hospital for the purpose of being given medical treatment for a mental disorder. If, 'but for' treatment of their physical disorder, then the person with the (pre-existing) mental disorder would not be detained then they are eligible under DoLS (*GJ* v. *the Foundation Trust*) and not a mental health patient as not within the scope of the MHA.

MHA/MCA interface

Choosing between the MHA and MCA was tested in *AM* v. *South London and Maudsley NHS Foundation Trust and the Secretary of State for Health*, where the judgment emphasised that only where a patient lacks capacity to consent to admission and treatment in a psychiatric hospital, and is not objecting to both aspects of care, is there a choice between the two regimes, in which case it is for the decision makers to determine which regime offers the least restrictive way of achieving the care and treatment objectives for that particular patient.

The confirmation from *Cheshire West* that deprivation of liberty can take place in a person's home and in other community settings has resulted in increased pressures on the Courts as an application to the Court of Protection (CoP) must take place in all such cases. A resultant '*re X* procedure' aims to streamline this process by a new CoP application form and a new practice direction (as of November 2014) but the Court of Appeal has cast doubt on the process (*Re X (Court of Protection Procedure)*) and the procedure remains controversial in its ability to satisfactorily comply with the ECHR.

In *Re SRK*, SRK suffered a brain injury as a result of a road traffic accident. He subsequently required 24-hour care (funded by the compensation payment, as was the purchase of an adapted bungalow). The continuous supervision and control, his lack of freedom to leave and his lack of capacity to consent to the care arrangements fulfilled the acid test.

However, the care was arranged by a case manager and provided by private carers, and the accommodation and care costs were privately funded and administered by a financial (court appointed) deputy, all without any input from the local authority. At issue was whether his confinement was attributable to the State, directly or indirectly, so as to engage Article 5. Charles J found in that case that the State was indirectly responsible for 'private' deprivations of liberty arising out of arrangements made by deputies administering personal injury payments.

The Secretary of State for Justice (SSJ) appealed but it was dismissed in *SSJ v. Staffordshire CC & Ors.* Sir Terence Atherton, Master of the Rolls (MR) in the Court of Appeal stated that 'Absent the making of a welfare order by the CoP, there are insufficient procedural safeguards against arbitrary detention in a purely private care regime' (echoing Lady Hale's statement that deprivation of liberty 'must mean the same for everyone'). In essence, wherever the state is, or ought to be, aware of a person being deprived of their liberty, it needs to ensure that deprivation is authorised. In the current DoLS framework, this requires authority from the Court of Protection under the *Re X* procedure.

That judge also noted that one of the unforeseen consequences of this ruling is that, where costs cannot be borne through (factoring in) a compensation award, 'it does come dangerously close to suggesting that people should pay for the privilege of having their detention authorised, to comply with the State's obligations'.

And while the essential tenets of the early Code of Practice guidance[8] remain the same, continuous development in case law has broadened the scope. The courts have confirmed for example that the use of covert medication constitutes an element of deprivation of liberty in *AG v. BMBC and SNH*, and that community treatment orders (CTO) and requirements set out in the care plan can, in certain situations, be considered a deprivation of liberty (*AG v. BMBC and SNH*).

In *AG v. BMBC and SNH*, it was accepted that covert medication is an interference with the right to respect for private life under Article 8 of the ECHR, and such treatment must be administered in accordance with law that guarantees proper safeguards against arbitrariness. Administering treatment to a person who cannot give informed consent and who is also not even passively accepting it when offered (hence the requirement for it to be given covertly) is also potentially a restriction contributing to the objective factors creating a deprivation of liberty within the meaning of Article 5 of the Convention as aspects of continuous supervision and control.

The Court discharged a DoLS for a patient in whom the main risk factor was of harm to others in *P v. A Local Authority* but in *N v. A Local Authority*, Justice Peter Jackson conformed to a liberal interpretation of harm to self by including the consequences to that person if the risk to others materialised. Is this a disingenuous balancing of harm to self (consequent only from infliction of harm to others) in the context of best interests, necessity and proportionality where a person suffers from a 'paedophiliac disorder'?

Deprivation of Liberty Safeguards: the future

These recent case law developments have served to modify our understanding of the 'Holy Grail' search for what constitutes a deprivation of liberty within the meaning of Article 5 HRA but the challenges highlighted in such cases serve to underline the parallel challenges of health and social care professionals in appropriately complying with the law, and in providing appropriate protection for society's most vulnerable citizens, with an additional challenge that full compliance with *Cheshire West* as it currently stands would require 2% of the entire budget of NHS England, according to an impact assessment carried out by the Law Commission (Mental Capacity and Deprivation of Liberty, 2017).

Even before *Cheshire West*, the Lords Select Committee on the MCA published a detailed report in March 2014 (Mental Capacity (amendment) Bill) concluding that the DoLS were 'not fit for purpose' and recommended that they be replaced. They felt that the DoLS do not protect individuals in the way Parliament had intended. The Department of Health then asked the Law Commission to review the DoLS (the latter set up in 1965 for the purpose of promoting the reform of the law) and they subsequently published their long-awaited review in March 2017 with a set of 47 recommendations (including that of replacing the DoLS as a matter of urgency) and a draft Bill (replacing the DoLS in its entirety), and running to 259 pages in total (Mental Capacity and Deprivation of Liberty, 2017). It applies to England and Wales only.

The Mental Capacity (Amendment) Bill and liberty protection safeguards

In response, the Government introduced the Mental Capacity (Amendment) Bill [HL] 2017–2019 in the House of Lords on 3 July 2018.[9] The Bill, published on 4 July 2018, accepts many of the recommendations but not others. The Department of Health in January 2019 announced that "Our Bill will reform a broken system and ensure vulnerable people have quicker access to legal protections by simplifying the process and minimising duplication, without compromising essential safeguards" (Guardian, 2019).

The reform of the DoLS seeks to introduce a simpler process, involving families and giving quicker access to assessments, allowing the NHS rather than local authorities to make decisions about their patients, end the current need for repeat assessments (and authorisations when a person moves from hospital, to home, to an ambulance) as part of their overall care (Department of Health, 2018).

A new Schedule AA1 Liberty Protection Safeguards (LPS) proposed in the Bill will replace DoLS. This is to avoid the negative connotations associated with the term deprivation of liberty. In using the language of 'necessary and proportionate' instead of 'best interests' to decide whether an individual should be cared for in circumstances that amount to a deprivation of liberty, and considered at the care planning stage for that individual, the Commission report and Bill have sought to address concerns that the 'best interests' assessment tended to act as a mere 'rubber stamp.' This is because currently decisions have often already been taken by a care team via the urgent authorisation procedure (allowing self-authorisation for seven days) meaning that assessments are in effect after the event.

In the report, and the Bill (in its final format), there is no provision for hospitals or care homes to issue themselves with urgent authorisations, and the Bill replaces the urgent authorisation with a statutory authority to deprive a person of their liberty temporarily in urgent situations Section 4B MCA will be amended so as to provide express authority for a person to take steps to deprive another person of their liberty if four conditions are met. Broadly speaking, section 4B will provide authority to take steps to deprive a person of their liberty in three circumstances: to enable life-sustaining treatment or to prevent a serious deterioration in their health, and also in situations where steps are being taken to obtain authorisation, or where a decision is being sought from the Court of Protection regarding authority to deprive a person of their liberty. Following a considerable level of debate in the "ping-pong" stage of the Bill's passage through both Houses, both Houses agreed to final amendments on the text of the Bill on 24.4.19 and it now therefore merely awaits the final stage of Royal Assent before it becomes law. No date has yet been set for this[10].

During the final debate in the House of Lords on 24.4.19, Baroness Murphy expressed disquiet stating that both Houses had allowed the Bill " to disintegrate into a sprawling, all-encompassing bit of a nightmare. the procedures may be simpler, we have cut out one layer of bureaucracy but we have allowed these provisions to be extended even further than Cheshire West. . .pursuing people in their own homes"[10].

The unforeseen complexity that came with DoLS in deciding in select cases whether the DoLS or MHA was the appropriate authority to use (Schedule 1A MCA dealing with this interface, described by Mostyn J in *An NHS Trust* v. *A* as 'a veritable smorgasbord of double negatives and subordinate clauses' and 'extreme opacity') was supposedly resolved by Law Commission proposals denying use of the MCA LPS for assessment and treatment of mental disorder, the report specifying that 'if arrangements [referred to in their draft Bill as 'mental health arrangements'] are to be carried out in hospital for the purpose of assessing, or providing medical treatment for a mental disorder, the LPS cannot be used to authorise these arrangements' (phrase in parenthesis added). 'The MHA should be used and objection will no longer be relevant. Treatment in such circumstances could be provided on an informal basis if there is a valid advance directive in place' which provides the informed consent. Law Commission proposals for LPS were that they would apply everywhere but 'in most cases, arrangements that involve the person being in hospital for assessment or treatment of a mental disorder cannot be authorised', effectively preventing the use of LPS in psychiatric hospitals. However, this has been dropped by the Bill in part 7 of schedule AA1, maintaining in most part the current status quo in this area. The Independent Review of the Mental Health Act, published 6.12.18[12], recommended that the law be amended so that the MCA can only be used in a psychiatric hospital where a person lacks capacity to consent to admission and treatment and it is clear they are not objecting, with the statutory definition for "objection" contained within the MCA, objection being the dividing line, and thus rejecting Law Commission proposals.

Key features of the Liberty Protection Safeguards (LPS) now include:

- Like DoLS (but contrary to the Law Commission's suggestion) they start at age 18. There is no statutory definition of a deprivation of liberty beyond that in the Cheshire West and Surrey Supreme Court judgement of March 2014 – the 'acid test'.
- Deprivations of liberty have to be authorised in advance by the 'responsible body'.
- For hospitals, be they NHS or private, the responsible body will be the 'hospital manager'.
- For arrangements under Continuing Health Care outside a hospital, the responsible body will be the local CCG (or Health Board in Wales).

- In all other cases – such as in care homes, supported living schemes (including for self-funders) – the responsible body will be the local authority.
- For the responsible body to authorise any deprivation of liberty, it needs to be clear that:

    The person who is the subject of the arrangements lacks the capacity to consent to the arrangements.

    The person has a mental disorder.

    The arrangements are necessary to prevent harm to the cared-for person and proportionate in relation to the likelihood and seriousness of harm to the cared-for person.

    Notably, in contrast to Law Commission proposals, there is no reference to the necessity and proportionality being judged either by reference to the risk of harm to the person themselves or by the risk of harm to others, the Government not seeking to reverse an amendment introduced in Lords tightening the definition solely to risk of harm to the person themselves[13].

- To determine this, the responsible body must consult with the person and others, to understand what the person's wishes and feelings about the arrangements are.
- An individual from the responsible body, but not someone directly involved in the care and support of the person subject to the care arrangements, must conclude if the arrangements meet the three criteria above (lack of capacity; mental disorder; necessity and proportionality).
- Where it is clear, or reasonably suspected, that the person objects to the care arrangements, then a more thorough review of the case must be carried out by an Approved Mental Capacity Professional.
- Where there is a potential deprivation of liberty in a care home, the Bill suggests the care home managers should lead on the assessments of capacity, and the judgement of necessity and proportionality, and pass their findings to the local authority as the responsible body. This aspect of the Bill generated some negative comment, with people feeling that there was insufficient independent scrutiny of the proposed care arrangements. This has been resolved in the final legislative debate, with a requirement for the responsible body to decide on whether it is confident that it is appropriate for the care home Manager to carry out these functions, prior to any authorisation, to resolve concerns of potential conflicts of interest in care homes (and this also applies to independent hospitals where a conflict of interest may arise)[11].
- Safeguards once a deprivation is authorised include regular reviews by the responsible body and the right to an appropriate person or an IMCA to represent a person and protect their interests.
- As under DoLS, a deprivation can be for a maximum of one year initially. Under LPS, this can be renewed initially for one year, but subsequent to that for up to three years.
- Again, as under DoLS, the Court of Protection will oversee any disputes or appeals.

The Law Commission identified a current narrow focus on Article 5 HRA in DoLS with little consideration of Article 8 HRA (the right to respect for privacy, family life … correspondence), recommending, therefore, a reform of the MCA to make more explicit a duty to consider such rights and improve decision-making, with greater weight accorded to determining ascertainable wishes, past and present, and, when these are not followed, a written record by decision makers as to why not. This reflected the Select Committee Report (House of Lords Select Committee on the Mental Capacity Act; UN Convention on the Rights of Persons with Disabilities; ECHR Convention for the Protection of Human

Rights and Fundamental Freedoms) that highlighted 'best interests' decisions regularly failing to give any weight to or to prioritise the person's wishes and feelings, as in *Neary (Hillingdon LB* v. *Neary)*, which also confirmed that DoLS cannot be used to remove a person from the family or prevent return to that family (protected by Article 8 HRA rights).

While 'best interests' is the cornerstone of the current system, the Law Commission proposed a simplified version of 'best interests' assessments but one which explicitly puts extra weight on the person's wishes and feelings. As has been noted in *N* v. *ACCG and others*, in reality a choice is often not available between different care options because the commissioning body will only fund one option, so a 'best interests' principle that sets out choices may be unrealistic in practice. The other reason that the Law Commission proposed the abandonment of 'best interests' is that it cannot be in a person's best interests to be deprived of their liberty where only required due to risk of harm to others, which is permitted by Strasbourg jurisprudence, but not by the MCA. The focus on the person's wishes and feelings has been dropped but will be addressed in the new Code of Practice that will accompany the legislation.

Additionally, on 24.4.19 agreement was reached as follows; "Amendments 25B and 25C state that after authorising arrangements, the responsible body must, without delay, arrange for a copy of the authorisation record to be given or sent. If the responsible body has not done this within 72 hours of the arrangements being authorised, it must review and record why not. The Government recognise the importance of providing people with information. We amended the Bill in the other place to clarify that people should be informed of their rights under the liberty protection safeguards process and provided with a copy of their authorisation record"[10]. However, LPS, unlike deprivation of liberty safeguards, does not provide authorisation to restrict a person's contact with other persons.

Section 5 MCA defence

But despite its commitment to abolish legislation that is 'overly bureaucratic', Law Commission proposals have recommended that a Section 5 MCA 'defence' that ('does not incur any liability in relation to the act' will not be available to professionals who fail to record decisions about moving a person to longer-term care and/or restrict their contact with others, provide serious medical treatment, administer covert medication or medication against a person's wishes, and in all these situations fail to demonstrate that the set of seven principles have been followed.

These include how the professional establishes a lack of capacity, and why they believe capacity is lacking, how they support the person to make their own decision, how they establish that the decision is in their 'best interests' and what the person's wishes and feelings are in relation to the decision (and if not followed, why not), that the duty to appoint advocacy is complied with, and confirmation that the decision is not contrary to an advance decision, including valid advance consent to the arrangements that amounts to a deprivation of liberty, which means there is no deprivation of liberty. This point was raised in the Law Commission's consultation that preceded the report (i.e. that they determined that a person cannot however give up their article 5 rights), but it was confirmed by the Strasbourg court that a person can only be deprived of their liberty if they have not validly consented to it (the valid consent contained within the advance decision). The Law Commission's proposal to allow advance consent to confinement was not taken forward.

Notably, the tort of deprivation of liberty is not included in the current Bill[10].

The Bill would apply to those with a mental disorder.

Fluctuating capacity has posed a number of problems to date as there is no guidance in the current Code of Practice, especially where a deprivation of liberty must be terminated if a person regains capacity. The Law Commission proposal is that this remains relevant only if capacity is regained for a short time, but the Bill is silent on this with fluctuating capacity not addressed in the final Bill[10].

Law Commission proposals and the Bill propose that LPS will cut out duplication as authorisations will be able to move from one setting to another, the 'supervisory body' becomes the 'responsible body' (Figure 4.1), and there will be an extension of who is responsible for giving authorisations. This would henceforth include NHS managers (a means by which a common link is maintained between the commissioners of care and the authorisation of the deprivation of liberty that is necessary for that care provision), so that no longer will local authorities be responsible for the deprivation of liberty authorisations in hospital settings.

If the authorisation is required in a hospital, then the responsible body will be the 'hospital manager', in most cases the hospital Trust. If the proposed arrangements are funded via continuing healthcare (CHC) funding, the responsible body is the local commissioning group, and for all others (including so-called self-funders) the local authority. The Bill introduces a new special procedure for care homes that effectively devolves responsibility to them (the care home managers) for arranging assessments with safeguards already referred to.

Under the current system of DoLS the assessments are coordinated by a best interests assessor (BIA), who will be replaced in the new system by a new Approved Mental Capacity Professional (AMCP), a role similar to the Approved Mental Health Professionals (AMHPs) with the requirement for a 'best interests' assessment to be dropped. AMCPs will focus on the more serious cases where there is demonstrable objection. Their role will be to meet with the person, and consult others, before providing written approval (or not) for authorisation of the deprivation of liberty, to the responsible body. The AMCP role could be undertaken by the same professionals who currently train as BIAs and current BIAs could be transferred to this new role – but this is not clarified in the Bill, however, the person completing assessments will have appropriate skilled knowledge[11].

The pre-authorisation review

The Law Commission proposed that every case would have an independent review by a reviewer who is an employee of the responsible body, but who is not involved in the person's care (now referred to in the Bill as a 'pre-authorisation review'). But if there are concerns regarding the placement (including where the person is objecting to the proposed arrangements), then a referral is made instead to the AMCP. The 'pre-authorisation review' of the assessments must take place, to 'confirm that it is reasonable for the responsible body to conclude that the conditions for authorisation are met' by 'scrutinising the assessments'. Following approval for authorisation (by either the independent reviewer or the AMCP), the responsible body will produce an 'authorisation record' containing relevant details of the care arrangements that amount to the deprivation of liberty.

Authorisation

The change in wording in the Law Commission Report and the Bill is to fulfil the requirement that the person is assessed to lack capacity, not for the fact of the placement

The Liberty Protection Safeguards
Summary of steps

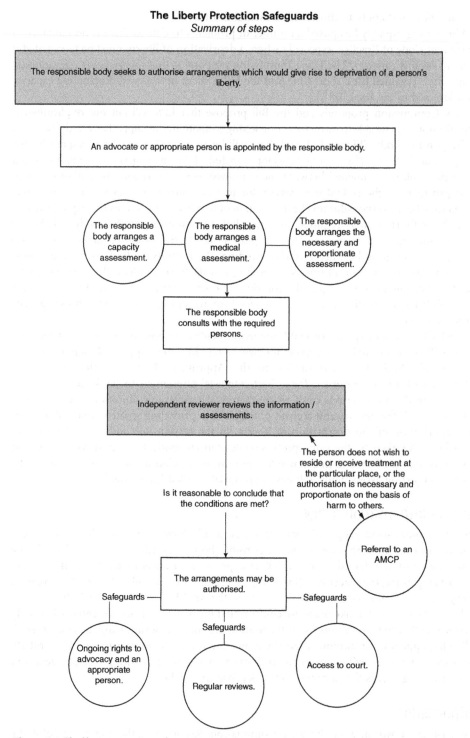

Figure 4.1 The liberty protection safeguards – summary of steps. © Crown copyright 2017. Full publication at https://s3-eu-west-2.amazonaws.com/lawcom-prod-storage-11jsxou24uy7q/uploads/2017/03/lc372_mental_capacity.pdf

itself, but for the 'arrangements' made including the elements of supervision and control, and lack of freedom to leave, the 'acid test'.

Currently, a deprivation of liberty authorisation merely authorises a deprivation of liberty, whereas the Law Commission proposed, and the Bill supports, that LPS would enable authorisations of particular 'arrangements' for a person's care and treatment insofar as the arrangements give rise to a deprivation of liberty, and, in comparison to DoLS, the capacity assessment for LPS will relate to the arrangements that constitute the deprivation of liberty. Authorisations could be given that also cover transportation, in addition to the care arrangements, and for care arrangements in different settings (for example care home environment and the person's own home), covering residence in more than one place. These specified care 'arrangements' themselves, including the transportation requirements associated with the care, are designed to cut bureaucracy and frequent repeat assessments. In effect, therefore, the provisions would allow for a new responsible body to make any changes to an existing authorisation so long as (a) there is consultation; (b) they are reasonable and (c) there is a review (either in advance or as soon as practicable thereafter). However, the Government's intention is that there are limits to what would otherwise be quite wide "portability" of authorisations, with Baroness Blackwood at the "ping-pong" stage in the Lords (26.2.19), stating that "[a]n authorisation can apply to different settings so that it can travel with a person but cannot be varied to apply to completely new settings once it has been made, as this would undermine Article 5."[10]

There is no specification in the Bill of the need for a medical doctor for assessment of mental disorder (akin to the Law Commission proposals), and the Bill (in contrast to the Law Commission proposals) does not specify the requirement of two assessors.

The potential widening of the group that can provide assessments envisaged by the Law Commission (and the Bill) is aimed at reducing costs, but what constitutes suitable experience and knowledge for such a role still remains unclear.

Time limits

The Bill, as in the proposals, permits authorisation for up to 12 months which can be renewed for up to a further 12 months, and can be renewed thereafter for up to three years (depending on the criteria for the care arrangements continuing to be met). An authorisation ceases at any time if the person regains capacity (for any considerable period) or is no longer suffering from a mental disorder or the arrangements are no longer necessary and proportionate.

Conditions

Conditions needing to be met will include therefore that the person lacks capacity to consent to the arrangements, the person has a mental disorder and the arrangements are necessary o prevent harm to the cared-for person and proportionate in relation to the likelihood and seriousness of harm to the cared-for person, the required consultation has been carried out, and an independent/'pre-authorisation' review has been carried out, and also (in certain cases only) the approval of a AMCP has been obtained. Changes in the person's condition or circumstances or a request by a person close to the person under LPS, or any detention under the MHA, will prompt a review by the responsible body.

The review process

Persons subject to LPS in the new Bill will have regular reviews of the arrangements authorised and the provision of an advocate or appropriate person to represent and support them during the initial process for authorisation and subsequently whilst subject to LPS. The duty to appoint someone to support the individual is similar to the current Relevant Person's Representative (RPR), or, where none is available, an advocate (IMCA). This 'appropriate person' cannot be a professional person involved in providing the care.

Guidance, hopefully, will be provided via a new Code of Practice as to the person specification for this role, including making it clear that the role of a supporter is to assist in decision-making whilst that of an independent advocate is to assist the person in making their views known.

UNCRPD considerations

Notable in the recommendations, but not in the Bill, were for this supported decision-making scheme to fulfil the 'aims and aspirations' of the United Nations Convention on the Rights of Persons with Disabilities (UNCRPD), which is applied in the ECtHR and referred to in *Cheshire West*. Of particular relevance are Articles 12 and 14, the former focusing on promoting that 'persons with disability enjoy legal capacity on an equal basis with others in all aspects of life'. The latter ensures liberty and security of the person and will be harder to effect but the principles of necessity and proportionality in all deprivation of liberty will hopefully minimise restrictions.

Advocacy

The Liberty Protection Safeguards in the Bill aim to deliver enhanced rights to advocacy, therefore, and give greater prominence to human rights considerations regarding whether the care arrangements that amount to a deprivation of liberty are necessary and proportionate.

Repeat assessments

As a means of providing for efficiency savings, reliance can be found in a recent capacity or medical assessment, as long as there is consideration of the purpose, any changes in the person's condition and the length of time since carried out. The Bill does not prescribe how reviews must be conducted but would include full participation of the person concerned, their family and professionals, and will be clarified possibly in a new Code of Practice.

Regulatory role

The CQC, and, in Wales, the Care and Social Services Inspectorate Wales and Healthcare Inspectorate Wales, would continue their monitoring role but their remit would change to include domestic settings, supported living and shared care environments. 'Light-touch' regulation is proposed in the additional environments, such as gathering information and interviewing people, with no recommendation to introduce any new powers to enter premises.

Fusion Law?

The report also raised the possibility of future 'fusion law' (a single legislative scheme governing non-consensual care or treatment of people suffering from physical and/or mental disorders whereby such care or treatment may only be given if the person lacks the capacity to consent) akin to that of the Mental Capacity (Northern Ireland) Act 2016 which incorporates mental health and capacity legislation into one statute.

Conclusion

In light of the above, some may wonder how our domestic law has strayed so far from other European countries that are also ECHR signatories (and therefore also bound by Strasbourg judgments). DoLS is a Convention violation in all of them under the same principles, and the perception of supervision and control may be very different to that of confinement, but *Cheshire West* disagrees. One of the appellants in that case was being provided with 1:1 support for 98 hours per week to enable him to leave his care environment and take part in social activities that any person without his level of need for care would enjoy. The continuous supervision and control could be interpreted as a means of *protecting* his right to liberty and freedom, and preventing confinement.

For those of us working in the health and social care sector, the DoLS have provoked a lot of anxiety and at times despair in trying to unravel different case law interpretations and in keeping up to date with ongoing changes as they emerge. The Commission report and newly published Bill in my view do nothing to allay those fears, with many key roles, responsibilities and principles (including a widely hoped for definition of what constitutes a deprivation of liberty) remaining undefined and therefore unclear. The heated debates during the ping-pong stage of the Bill, that centred on the need for a statutory definition of what constitutes a DoL (and what that definition would be) are supposedly resolved by relegating it to the Code of Practice. To ensure that the meaning will be regularly reviewed, an approved amendment incorporates a duty to review the definition to ensure it is kept up to date with evolving case law and that there will be a report of that review laid before Parliament within three years of the measures coming into force, and subsequently every 5 years[10].

The duty to be consistent with ECtHR (principle-based) law and our own domestic (case-based and statute (MHA/MCA)) law appears to require a vexatious squeezing of the square peg of ECHR deprivation of liberty into the round hole of the combined domestic MCA/MHA case law. Is this Bill, soon to be given Royal Assent, or fusion law our best hope for the future?

References

Bowcott, O. (2019) Mental capacity changes give care homes too much power, critics say. Guardian News Article. https://www.theguardian.com/uk-news/2019/jan/17/mental-health-changes-england-wales-give-care-homes-too-much-power-government-warned

Crews, M., Garry, D., Phillips, C., Wong, A., Troke, B., Ruck Keene, A. & Danbury, C. (2014) Deprivation of liberty in intensive care. The Intensive Care Society.

Department of Health Guidance (2015) *Response to the Supreme Court Judgment/Deprivation of Liberty Safeguards,* Department of Health, 22 October.

Department of Health (2018) *New law introduced to protect vulnerable people in care,* Department of Health, 3 July 2018

ECHR Convention for the Protection of Human Rights and Fundamental Freedoms (Rome 1950).

Mental Capacity Act 2005. House of Lords Select Committee on the Mental Capacity Act: Report of session 2013–2014: Mental Capacity Act 2005: Post-legislative Scrutiny [2014] HL 139 paragraph 32.

Mental Capacity Act 2005. Deprivation of Liberty Safeguards (England) Annual report 2014–2015. Health and Social Care information centre.

Mental Capacity and Deprivation of Liberty, Law Commission no. 372. HMSO 2017.

Mental Capacity (amendment) Bill [HL] 2017–2019.

Report of the Chief Coroner to the Lord Chancellor, third annual report 2015–2016.

UN Convention on the Rights of Persons with Disabilities (adopted 13 December 2006, entered into force 3 May 2008) 2515 UNTS 3 (CRPD).

Case law

AM v. South London and Maudsley NHS Foundation Trust and the Secretary of State for Health [2013] UKUT 0365 (AAC).

Cheshire West and Chester Council v. P [2014] UKSC 19 [2014] MHLO 16.

GJ v. the Foundation Trust [2009] EWHC 2972 (fam) [2010].

Guzzardi v. Italy [1980] 3 EHRR 333 (app No 7367/76).

HL v. UK [2004] 40 EHRR 761.

Liverpool City Council, Nottinghamshire County Council, LB of Richmond upon Thames and Shropshire Council v. SSH.

N v. ACCG and others [2017] UKSCC 22.

N v. A Local Authority [2016] EWCOP 47.

Neary (Hillingdon LB v. Neary) [2011] EWHC 1377 (COP) [2011] 4 All ER 584.

NHS Trust and others v. FG [2014] EWCOP 30.

NHS Trust I v. G [2015] 1 WLR 1984.

P v. A Local Authority [2015] COP no 12715633.

R (Ferreira) v. HM Senior Coroner for Inner South London and others [2017] EWCA Civ 31.

Re SRK [2016] EWCOP 27.

Re X (Court of Protection Procedure) [2015] EWCA Civ 599.

SSJ v. Staffordshire CC & Ors [2016] EWCA Civ 1317.

Storck v. Germany 61603/00 [2005] ECHR 406.

Wintwerp v. Netherlands 6301/73 [1979] ECHR 4.

Notes

1 www.legislation.gov.uk/ukpga/2005/9/schedule/A1 (accessed 11.7.2017).

2 www.mentalhealthlaw.co.uk/Mental_disorder_no_longer_split_into_separate_classifications (accessed 6.8.2017).

3 MCA Code of practice at www.gov.uk/government/publications/mental-capacity-act-code-of-practice (accessed 6.8.2017) and DoLS Code of Practice, Ministry of Justice Mental Capacity Act 2005: *Deprivation of Liberty Safeguards: code of practice to supplement the Main Mental Capacity Act 2005 Code of Practice* (2008).

4 www.gov.uk/government/uploads/system/uploads/attachment_data/file/556032/Deprivation_of_Liberty_Safeguards_England_Annual_Report_2015-16.pdf (accessed 9.7.2017).

5 Ibid.

6 assets.publishing.service.gov.uk/government/uploads/system/uploads/attachment_data/file/715224/death-certification-reforms-government-response.pdf; www.lawcom.gov.uk/project/mental-capacity-and-deprivation-of-liberty/ (accessed 8.8.2018).

7 MCA Code of practice at https://www.gov.uk/government/publications/mental-capacity-act-code-of-practice (accessed 6.8.17) and DoLS Code of Practice, Ministry of Justice Mental Capacity Act 2005: *Deprivation of Liberty Safeguards: code of practice to supplement the Main Mental Capacity Act 2005 Code of Practice* (2008).

8 Ibid.

9 www.brownejacobson.com/health/training-and-resources/legal-updates/2018/06/the-death-of-dols-the-liberty-protection-safeguards-are-before-parliament-now (accessed 8.8.2018).

10   hansard.parliament.uk/lords/2019-04-24/debates/9559EF20-61B3-4AD9-8A68-9195A845FE1C/Debate (accessed 26.04.2019).

11   www.gov.uk/government/publications/modernising-the-mental-health-act-final-report-from-the-independent-review (accessed 26.4.19).

12   www.mentalcapacitylawandpolicy.org.uk/lps-where-are-we-and-where-are-we-going/ (accessed 26.4.19).

13   www.scie.org.uk/files/mca/directory/dols/cbp-8466.pdf?res=true (accessed 26.4.19).

Mental Capacity Act Application: Hospital Settings

Elizabeth Fistein

Introduction

Case study 5.1   Peter

Peter is a 63-year-old man who has a long history of bipolar affective disorder. He lives alone in his own flat, and has a network of caring family and friends. He takes lithium as a mood stabiliser, but nonetheless experiences manic episodes every two years or so. During those periods, Peter believes that he is immortal and that he can cure illnesses and injuries through the power of his mind. He becomes irritable and disinhibited, and can get into fights which put him and others in danger. These episodes of mania have always been successfully treated with antipsychotic medication. Peter has also recently developed angina, and he is prescribed atenolol and simvastatin.

The purpose of the Mental Capacity Act can be thought of as follows: a means of providing legal justification for actions in connection with a person, which would normally require the consent of that person, when it is not possible to obtain consent on the grounds that the person lacks the decision-making capacity to give or withhold legally valid consent. In other words, if a healthcare professional needs to do something, which would normally be unlawful if they did not gain the patient's consent, but the patient is unable to give consent, then the Mental Capacity Act provides a framework.

In hospital settings, there are three main areas of activity which would normally require the consent of the patient: providing medical treatment, sharing information which could identify a patient with a third party and providing care which requires the patient to remain in hospital. In this chapter, the application of the Mental Capacity Act to common scenarios that arise in each of these three areas is outlined. Peter's case is used as an example of the kinds of situation that may arise.

Medical treatment

Case study 5.1   (cont.)

Peter experiences early warning signs of a manic episode and he agrees to attend his local Accident and Emergency Department. After waiting a couple of hours to see a psychiatrist, he becomes extremely agitated, strips off and runs around the department trying to hit anyone who gets in his way. He is offered oral medication (lorazepam) to help him to feel calmer, but he knocks the tablets out of the nurse's hand.

In this situation, urgent treatment for Peter's mental health condition is required to prevent him from inadvertently injuring himself or anyone else. As he is refusing oral medication, it may be necessary to administer an intra-muscular injection for rapid tranquillisation. Under normal circumstances, Peter's consent would be required and administering an injection against his will would amount to unlawful assault. To determine whether there is a legal justification for treating without consent, it is necessary to consider the purpose and urgency of the treatment, the setting in which it will be given, and the patient's decision-making capacity.

Purpose: Rapid tranquillisation is medical treatment for a mental disorder. Potentially, the Mental Health Act provides justification for treatment, and should be used in preference to the Mental Capacity Act, if this is practical. However, the question of whether the Mental Health Act will apply depends upon how quickly treatment is needed and where the patient is.

Urgency: The treatment is needed immediately.

Setting: Peter is in the Emergency Department.

If the Mental Health Act is to provide justification for treatment without consent, an assessment will have to be carried out by two doctors and an Approved Mental Health Professional, and the patient will have to be admitted to a mental health ward under Section 2 or 3. This is not clinically appropriate under these circumstances. Therefore, use of the Mental Capacity Act should be considered. The first step is to assess capacity.

All adults are presumed to have capacity to make treatment decisions, unless a capacity assessment demonstrates otherwise (MCA, Section 1(2)). In a situation like this, any doctor should be able to swiftly assess capacity by observing Peter's abnormal behaviour and asking him one or two quick questions. It is very likely that this assessment will result in the conclusion that Peter lacks capacity to consent to medical treatment at this time. If this is the case, a timely determination of best interests is required.

The Mental Capacity Act only authorises others to act in the best interests of the person who lacks capacity, not in the interests of anyone else (MCA, Section 1(5)). In Peter's case, it may be in his interests to receive rapid tranquillisation in order to prevent him from injuring himself, or to prevent him from behaving in an aggressive way, which, if he had capacity to make the decision, he would wish to have treatment to prevent. This may mean that treatment is in his best interests. The safety of others is not, in itself, a factor.

It is possible that a patient's best interests can be served by the use of restraint using medical treatment. The law does not distinguish between physical restraint and pharmacological restraint by sedation. Where restraint is used, in addition to being in the patient's best interests, it must be necessary to prevent harm and be proportionate to the likelihood and seriousness of that harm.

Practical advice

- For acutely disturbed patients in accident and emergency (A&E) or general hospital wards, the Mental Health Act may not provide a suitable framework for emergency psychiatric treatment, such as rapid tranquillisation, and use of the Mental Capacity Act should be considered.

- Do not presume that an adult lacks capacity or that treatment must be in his or her best interests. When a patient is acutely disturbed, capacity can be assessed very swiftly, on the basis of behavioural symptoms and ability to engage in discussion about treatment.

- Any decision about the patient's best interests should always be tested with the question: is there a less restrictive way to meet their best interests?

Case study 5.1 (*cont.*)

Peter is assessed and admitted to the local psychiatric unit under Section 3 of the Mental Health Act. After a couple of days, his agitation settles considerably and he usually accepts the tablets prescribed for him (olanzapine, plus his regular lithium, atenolol and simvastatin). However, he continues to believe that he is immortal and does not need medication because he can cure himself. He tells the nurses that he knows they know this too, and this is why they are just giving him these sugar pills. Sometimes he flatly refuses the medication, and the nurses tell him he must have it and sit with him until he accepts it.

Purpose: Once Peter is detained in hospital under the Mental Health Act, his consent is not required for *medical treatment* for his *mental disorder* (MHA, Section 63). However, Section 63 does not provide any justification for the treatment of *physical disorder* without consent, unless it is a direct cause or consequence of the patient's mental disorder. As an adult, Peter has the right to refuse his atenolol and simvastatin unless he lacks the capacity to make a decision about taking them, in which case the nurses are justified in coercing him to take the tablets, provided the treatment is in his best interests.

Capacity: Peter cannot be presumed to lack capacity simply because he is detained under the Mental Health Act (MCA, Section 2(3)(b)). However, his beliefs about his own immortality and ability to cure himself, and that the tablets he is being offered are sugar pills, suggest that, regardless of whether or not he accepts the medication, he is unable to understand, weigh and use information relevant to the decision to take medication, which amounts to incapacity to make this decision (MCA, Section 3).

Practical advice

- The Mental Capacity Act may be needed for aspects of treatment aimed at treating physical disorder, even when other aspects of treatment aimed at treating mental disorder are justified by Section 63 of the Mental Health Act.
- The condition which makes detention under the Mental Health Act necessary may also impair ability to understand, retain, weigh and use information relevant to a decision about treatment for a physical co-morbidity. If this is the case, the Mental Capacity Act provides justification for treatment, provided it is in the patient's best interests.

Case study 5.1 (*cont.*)

Peter begins to recover over the course of the next fortnight. He stops believing he is immortal and can cure himself, and regains his insight into the need for treatment for his mental and physical health. However, he becomes increasingly reluctant to take atenolol and his named nurse asks the Core Trainee in Psychiatry working on his ward to have a word with him. Peter explains to the junior doctor that he knows that the atenolol will reduce his risk of having a heart attack, but he hates the side effects (fatigue and erectile dysfunction) so much, he would rather take his chances and stop the medication.

As stated above, Peter cannot be presumed to lack capacity simply because he is detained under the Mental Capacity Act (MCA, Section 2(3)(b)). As long as he is able to understand, retain, weigh and use the relevant information, and communicate his decision, he is free to make any decision he wishes about his physical health. His decision does not have to be wise or well-reasoned; it is his decision-making capacity or ability, not the decision he makes, that is relevant (MCA, Section 1(4)).

Capacity: In this situation, Peter appears to understand the risks and benefits of continuing to take atenolol and of discontinuing the treatment. This means he does not lack the relevant decision-making capacity, and his refusal of treatment must be respected.

Practical advice

- Be aware of the risk of being swayed by your own evaluation of the wisdom of a patient's decision when assessing capacity: always apply the MCA's test of capacity.
- Unwise decisions by people who are able to understand, retain, weigh and use information relevant to the decision, and to communicate their decision, must be respected. This applies regardless of the presence or absence of mental ill-health.

Case study 5.1 *(cont.)*

Peter recovers sufficiently to return home. A few days later, he experiences severe chest pain and calls 999. He is rushed to hospital with a suspected myocardial infarction. After an ECG and blood tests confirm the diagnosis, coronary angioplasty and stent insertion is recommended. The cardiologist notes that Peter has recently been 'sectioned' and doubts he will be able to give consent for this procedure.

Purpose: Coronary angioplasty is a potentially life-saving treatment for Peter's physical condition.

Urgency: This is a medical emergency and treatment is needed as soon as possible.

Capacity: Capacity is decision specific. It is possible for a patient to have capacity to make one decision whilst simultaneously lacking capacity to make another, more complex, decision. In contrast to the decision to take atenolol, the decision to undergo an invasive procedure, such as coronary angioplasty, is more complex and may require a higher degree of ability to comprehend and analyse information. However, Peter's recent status as a detained patient is not relevant to the assessment of his capacity – it must be based upon his ability to make this decision at this point in time. A person is not to be regarded as unable to understand the information relevant to a decision if he is able to understand an explanation of it given to him in a way that is appropriate to his circumstances (using simple language, visual aids or any other means) (MCA, Section 3(2)).

Practical advice

- Beware of making unjustified assumptions about capacity on the basis of a particular diagnosis: always apply the MCA's test of capacity (MCA, Section 3).
- Where there are concerns about a patient's decision-making capacity, remember to assess their capacity to make the relevant decision, at the relevant point in time.

Sharing information

Treatment without consent is, in the absence of another justification, assault. Similarly, sharing information about a patient's health without their consent is, in the absence of another justification, a breach of confidentiality. There are numerous potential justifications for breaching confidentiality, discussion of which is beyond the scope of this book. However, the Mental Capacity Act does apply to some decisions about information sharing.

Case study 5.1 *(cont.)*

Unfortunately, the angioplasty does not go according to plan and Peter suffers a stroke. He is transferred to ITU. Peter's sister, Louise, is concerned that he has not been answering his telephone and contacts his neighbours who inform her that Peter was taken to hospital in an ambulance. Louise telephones the hospital to ask what has happened to her brother. The staff nurse who takes the call is reluctant to tell her anything, as she knows she must respect patient confidentiality.

Healthcare professionals generally take their duty of confidentiality very seriously and with good reason: it is an important factor in maintaining the trust of the public. Nonetheless, there is usually no need to withhold information from concerned relatives. In most cases, hospital staff will ask their patients for consent to inform their loved ones of their condition and progress, and only decline to answer questions if consent was not forthcoming. However, it will not always be possible to seek consent, for example, if the patient was admitted unconscious in an emergency or if they had a pre-existing condition such as advanced dementia. Under those circumstances, where the patient is assessed as lacking capacity to make a decision about sharing information with their loved ones, hospital staff must determine whether sharing this information would be in the patient's best interests. It may be in the patient's interests to share information if it enables a friend or relative to better support their recovery, or if this would be in accordance with what is known of the patient's past and present wishes and feelings, and the beliefs and values that may have influenced their decision, if they had the capacity to make one.

Practical advice

- Wherever possible, ask patients if you can share information about their condition and progress with loved ones, and respect their wishes if there is particular information that they do not want to be disclosed, or someone they do not want information to be shared with.
- When there are concerns about a patient's ability to make a decision about disclosure, assess their capacity to make this decision and, if necessary, act in their best interests (not the interests of their relative). Often, this will involve sharing some information.

Case study 5.1 *(cont.)*

Whilst Peter is recovering from the stroke, he has difficulty swallowing and a decision has to be made about using a percutaneous endoscopic gastrostomy (PEG) for clinically assisted nutrition and hydration. He has cognitive impairment and a dense aphasia which are impairing his ability to make and communicate complex decisions.

When determining the best interests of a patient who lacks the capacity to make a particular decision about treatment, healthcare professionals should, where practicable, consult with 'anyone engaged in caring for the person or interested in his welfare' as to what would be in the patient's best interests (MCA, Section 4(7)(b)). Their views must be taken into account, but they are not determinative.

In this example, if Louise is involved in caring for Peter or is interested in his welfare (as seems likely), the doctors should discuss the possibility of inserting a PEG with her. This will, inevitably, involve disclosing some information about Peter's health – why he needs a PEG, and what the likely risks and benefits of this procedure are. Disclosing this information will not amount to an unlawful breach of confidentiality, because the disclosure is mandated by the statutory requirement to consult with Louise.

Practical advice

- If a patient lacks capacity to make a healthcare decision, doctors are, when practicable and appropriate, obliged to consult, and take into account the views of anyone involved in caring for the patient or interested in their welfare.
- This will involve the disclosure of some information about the patient's condition, so that the person being consulted can understand why the treatment has been suggested.

Providing care

> **Case study 5.1** *(cont.)*
>
> Whilst Peter is recovering in the ITU, he is confined to bed and requires constant supervision. He remains quite confused, with fluctuating levels of consciousness and cannot understand much of what is happening to him. His treating team are aware of his history of mental ill-health, and discuss whether they need to apply for DoLS authorisation.

As discussed in Chapter 4 on deprivation of liberty, the Supreme Court judgment in *Cheshire West* clarified the definition of a deprivation of liberty. Where lack of capacity to consent to arrangements for care and treatment, continuous supervision and control, and a lack of freedom to leave are all present together, the test is met. However, in the more recent case *Ferreira* v. *Coroner of Inner South London* (2017), the Court of Appeal decided that 'any deprivation of liberty resulting from the administration of life-saving treatment to a person falls outside Article 5(1) [the right to liberty] ... so long as [it is] rendered unavoidable as a result of circumstances beyond the control of the authorities and is necessary to avert a real risk of serious injury or damage, and [is] kept to the minimum required for that purpose ... The treatment must be given in good faith and is materially the same treatment as would be given to a person of sound mind with the same physical illness.'

In our example, Peter's care arrangements might, on the face of it, appear to meet the criteria for a DoLS authorisation: he is over 18, has a mental disorder, is subject to continuous supervision and control, is not free to leave, lacks capacity to consent to the arrangement, is not liable to detention under the Mental Health Act (due to the setting where his treatment is taking place – ITU, and the purpose of that treatment – to enable him to recover from a stroke), the deprivation of liberty is taking place in his best interests, and an authorisation would not contradict or conflict with an advance decision to refuse treatment (MCA, Schedule A1).

However, following the decision in *Ferreira*, a DoLS authorisation would not be required. The 'not free to leave' element of the *Cheshire West* test requires that the patient is prevented from leaving by the detaining authority; the test is not satisfied when the reason the patient is not able to leave is their underlying medical condition.

Practical advice

- When a care plan appears to amount to a deprivation of liberty, but is not materially different to the care that would be offered to the patient if they had no mental disorder, there is no need for a DoLS referral.
- If, however, the care plan differs from that offered to other patients with the same physical health needs but without a mental disorder, then a DoLS referral is advisable.

Case study 5.1 *(cont.)*

Peter recovers his mobility but his cognitive capacity remains impaired, and he is transferred to a neuro-rehabilitation ward. His cognitive capacity deteriorates after two further cerebro-vascular events, and he is diagnosed with vascular dementia. Peter is unable to return home to his flat, and remains on the ward while a residential placement that can meet his needs is found. He is often confused, and, having wandered out of the hospital in his pyjamas one night, is kept under close observation and is guided away from the door when he tries to leave. He appears to accept the arrangement.

In this situation, by way of contrast, a DoLS authorisation may be required. Peter is over 18 years old, and now has two mental disorders: bipolar affective disorder and vascular dementia. He is subject to continuous supervision and control, is not free to leave, and still lacks capacity to consent to the arrangement. He is, on balance, probably not subject to detention under the Mental Health Act on two grounds: he is going along with the admission and care plan (making detention unnecessary) and he is not in hospital to receive medical treatment for either of his mental disorders – he is simply awaiting a place in a suitable care home. A patient awaiting placement in a care home because of physical health needs, who did not have vascular dementia, would, in all likelihood, not be prevented from leaving the ward in the same way Peter is. Provided the deprivation of liberty is found to be in his best interests, and not in conflict with an advance decision to refuse treatment, then it can be authorised.

Practical advice

- If the root cause of any loss of liberty is not the patient's physical condition, but restrictions imposed by the hospital because of the patient's mental disorder, then a patient who is subject to continuous supervision and control and is not free to leave is subject to a deprivation of liberty.
- Detention under the Mental Health Act should be considered, but if this is not appropriate, then a DoLS referral should be made.

Conclusion

There are a wide variety of situations experienced by adult patients in hospital where healthcare professionals are required to apply the Mental Capacity Act. The MCA is relatively easily understood and applied in the context of treating a physical health problem in a general hospital ward. The application is more complicated in contexts such as the treatment of mental disorder (where the Mental Health Act may provide an alternative legal justification for treatment without consent), and the treatment of a physical condition for a patient who has been detained for treatment of mental ill-health.

- Generally speaking, the MCA will be used for the treatment of physical conditions, whereas the MHA can only be used for the treatment of mental disorders (including physical conditions that directly cause, or are directly caused by, the mental disorder).
- However, the MCA can also be used for the treatment of mental disorders when it is not possible or appropriate to detain the patient under the MHA (e.g. when emergency psychiatric treatment is needed in accident and emergency, or for an informal psychiatric patient, and it is not possible to arrange detention under the MHA, or when short-term treatment is needed for a patient with delirium in a general hospital).

The MCA does not only apply to decisions about medical treatment, it may also apply to decisions about sharing information with a patient's loved ones and to care arrangements for patients with a mental disorder that amount to a deprivation of liberty (where these differ from the arrangements that would be in place for a patient without a mental disorder). The DoLS framework is complex, and is set to be replaced by new liberty deprivation safeguards in the near future. Healthcare professionals should keep up to date with developments, and seek expert advice if they are unsure of their legal obligations in any given case.

References

Mental Health Act 1983, as amended 2007.

Mental Capacity Act 2005.

Case law

Cheshire West and Chester Council v. P [2014] UKSC 19 [2014] MHLO 16.

R (Ferreira) v. HM Senior Coroner for Inner South London [2017] EWCA Civ 31, [2017] MHLO 2.

Mental Capacity Act Application: Social Care Settings

Michael Dunn and Anthony Holland

Introduction

Following the Mental Capacity Act (MCA) becoming law in 2005, and prior to its coming into force in 2007, there was a sustained effort to train support staff in the many social care settings where this new law was applicable. This training drive was necessary because, prior to the MCA, mental capacity law had evolved in the courts through consideration of a small number of cases that concerned serious medical treatments. These included the withdrawal of artificial nutrition and hydration (*Airedale NHS Trust* v. *Bland* [1993]), blood transfusion (*Re T* [1993]), tissue donation (*Re Y* [1997]) and the provision of experimental medication for terminal illness (*Simms* v. *Simms and another* (2003)). In line with the Law Commission's recommendations, the MCA extended the application of the law to 'all acts in connection with care or treatment' (MCA, Section 5), meaning that, overnight, social care settings and informal family care environments immediately fell within the scope of the legislation.

The Government's intention was that the new legislation, with its principles set out in Section 1, would be a radical and enabling law where the focus would be on involvement, inclusion and choice. The emphasis of the MCA's provisions is to do things *with* rather than *for* people who may have difficulties making decisions for themselves – an orientation towards person-centred care that aligned closely with the historical and philosophical trajectory of social care services. Yet, its primary purpose as legislation consists in its new regulatory requirements that determine when, and under what circumstances, care staff, who need to provide support to an adult, are permitted to make that decision on behalf of the adult concerned, when it would normally have been a decision for the adult to make for him/herself.

In first getting to grips with how to apply the MCA in social care settings, it is useful to consider the MCA from two standpoints. The first standpoint concerns the philosophy of care that underpins the legislation, and the second concerns the legal powers that it authorises – powers which can be particularly significant when the person being supported is acting in a manner that is potentially putting him/herself at risk. Specific issues dealt with by the MCA in social care settings concern adults' capacity to make decisions; uncertainty about how to conceptualise best interests; the safeguarding of adults' freedom to act within a supported environment and issues around the broader responsibilities that support staff have in planning their work and care interventions. In this chapter, we aim to show that the application of the MCA in these settings is particularly demanding given the general challenges faced by the social care sector, the heterogeneity of those being supported and the range of decisions that need to be made on a day-to-day basis – from the relatively minor to the potentially very serious.

Background: the changing landscape of social care services

The focus of social care policy has, over many years, moved away from hospital-based or institutional care to a much greater emphasis on home-based interventions that respect individual choice, and that broaden the availability of support options according to need. The social care landscape is now characterised by services that offer a few hours a week of home-based care, to supported living, to long-term residential care, typically in suburban home-like environments. Unlike in-patient healthcare, social care support is provided through a marketplace of services in which private and third-sector organisations bid for contracts, and the quality of care subsequently provided is monitored, in England and Wales, through periodic Care Quality Commission (CQC) inspections. This market system and the division between purchasers (commissioners) and providers of services, it was argued, would be best able to respond to changing needs and deliver high-quality support. However, there are increasing concerns that this system is dysfunctional and under-funded by local authorities. With increasing pressure on resources, the viability of individual social care providers and the system as a whole is at risk. Importantly, these changing circumstances are also relevant to the application of the MCA, and the propagation of its empowering principles.

In addition to the complex and changing service models that exist, it is also important to appreciate the heterogeneity and increasing complexity of need of those in receipt of these services. It is particularly those adults with disorders that have impacted on the functioning of the central nervous system, and/or have resulted in significant mental health needs, that come within the remit of social care services. This is because it is these adults who require care or support in numerous aspects of their personal and social lives, or because of more specific health needs. Examples include people with intellectual (learning) disabilities, enduring mental illness, an acquired brain injury or dementia. For some, the impairment or disability in question will have been life-long. For others, they may have developed a progressive disorder of the brain later in life. Some will experience life-long impairments that impact on their capacity to make any decisions, whilst others will have cognitive impairments or mental states that fluctuate over time. Changing demographics will also have a major impact on need, given the likely rise in age-related cognitive illnesses. Between 2012 and 2032, the population of 65–84-year-olds and those over 85, in the UK, is expected to increase by 39% and 106% respectively (King's Fund, 2012). Alongside improved survival rates of people with complex disabilities of childhood origin, and higher expectations placed on the quality of services provided, these trends are all likely to add to the complexity and pressure on the services concerned.

The MCA in social care practice: everyday decisions that need to be made

The MCA sits in the background of this complex and changing care landscape, providing the overarching legal framework to permit everyday care and treatment decisions to be made on behalf of others. In hospital settings, the decisions in question will in general be focused on the need for investigations and treatment. In contrast, in social care the decisions may be more nebulous and are likely to be concerned with a mixture of routine issues, including day-to-day decisions about what to eat, what to wear and what to do during the day. However, there will also be decisions that need to be made that are of great significance, and the outcomes of which have the potential for both benefit and harm to the person concerned. Examples of such potentially problematic decisions include moving between social care settings and the basic freedoms that the person will be able to enjoy in a different residential environment. Decisions around personal relationships and friendships can also be very challenging, particularly when there are concerns about exploitation and abuse, or when the person is engaging in behaviours that stand in stark contrast to the values or preferences they exhibited earlier in life. Those providing social care support also may be faced with what to do when there are concerns about a person's health and the person him/herself is refusing to do anything about it.

In all situations, those providing support should have a good relationship with the care recipient, and be appropriately supported themselves by senior colleagues to make decisions and take action in ways that address any legal, ethical or practical concerns that go beyond mere questions of mental capacity. During the course of providing support, it may, for example, become apparent that rather than being a question of cognitive understanding, the problem for the person is knowing how to deal interpersonally with 'friends' who are acting in an abusive manner, or are his/her only 'friends' in what is for him/her a lonely existence. Or, perhaps, the problem may be fear about going to the GP or the hospital following negative experiences of past health interventions. These are examples where the issue is not fundamentally about whether or not someone has the capacity to make a decision, rather it is the challenges in supporting a service user to negotiate relationships, or to manage anxiety, that staff need to attend to.

Care must also be taken to ensure that regulatory powers around mental capacity and substitute decision-making do not function to turn the value of empowerment on its head, seeing a judgement of capacity as foreclosing the possibility of providing further care and support interventions to the person. There have been recent examples portrayed in the media where a person in receipt of care has died for reasons that could have been prevented, but where it appears that nothing was done as the person was considered to have the capacity to make the relevant decision. This kind of situation shows that lying in the background of the MCA are ongoing ethical issues concerning, for example, how best to balance respect for choice against taking necessary steps to address potential harms. These issues will need to be addressed, regardless of whether the person is judged, legally, to have the capacity to make a decision for him/herself.

In cases like these, the issue of the person's capacity to make the relevant decision is certainly relevant. However, appropriate care also hinges on the quality of support provided: the relationship that staff have with the person concerned, and staff members' willingness to better understand the person's apparent refusal to negotiate harms and benefits in the social care environment, and then to act accordingly. In many circumstances, there will be systematic issues that will need to be addressed in social care in order to resolve these issues and to apply the MCA in ways that adhere to the overarching spirit of the legislation. The quality and expertise of support staff and particularly senior support staff, the availability or not of other expertise and the practicalities of lawful interventions in circumstances where those receiving care may have funding for only limited support, all need to be recognised as significant in this context.

Assessment of decision-making capacity in social care settings

The MCA is clear that the assessment of mental capacity, and an orientation towards care and support more generally, should start from presuming that the person is capable of autonomous decision-making. If there is doubt as to the person's capacity, in relation to a specific decision, this is to be determined by a two-stage test. The first stage is to determine whether or not the person has 'an impairment or disability of the brain or mind', and this diagnostic threshold will almost always apply in social care. The second stage requires a determination that, because of this impairment or disability and having provided the person with time and the necessary information in the most easy-to-digest format, the person is unable to understand, retain or use and weigh up the information and/or to communicate a choice.

We draw on three examples of people living in the community where there was uncertainty about capacity and where their behaviour had the potential to put them and/ or others at risk. These examples are:

- **Miss A** has a severe intellectual disability (ID). She receives intensive support in all day-to-day activities in a residential care home. She has been seen to be engaging in sexual touching with a male resident.
- **Mr B** had a severe traumatic brain injury as a teenager. Now 25, he is spending the money received from his insurance company in ways that his support workers consider are reckless.
- **Mrs C** has dementia. She is still living in her own house but behaving in ways that are beginning to put her increasingly at risk of harm. Her family are considering supporting her to re-locate to a residential care home but are concerned that this is not something that she would want.

First, social care staff need to be aware what information needs to be known and under-stood in order for the person to be judged to have the capacity to make a specific decision. Generally, this involves determining whether the person understands specific facts about the decision to be made – the so-called 'salient facts' (*LBJ* v. *RYJ & VJ* [2010]) – rather than the broader context or the wider implications associated with making the decision in a particular way. Thus, Mr B and Mrs C will be judged to understand the information, and use it and weigh it in making a decision, if they can give a coherent, reasoned account of the decision, and can reasonably foresee the consequences of it. Even if care staff do not agree with how Mr B and Mrs C are using or weighing up the information in making a decision with potentially negative consequences, this is irrelevant to the question of whether they can, in fact, use or weigh the information in the decision-making process. Also, Mr B and Mrs C do not need to be able to grasp and consider all potential risks associated with the decision. Nor do they need to take a considered view on the relationship between the decision and the harm that might result, in light of their personal values or preferences. A common feature of social care settings is the interface between (i) individual vulnerabil-ities, (ii) environmental circumstances, (iii) the demands of a particular decision-making task, (iv) a potential changing or fluctuating impairment in function and (v) the porous boundary between what might be a capacitous (but foolhardy) decision versus an incapa-citous decision. Those providing support will have to make difficult judgements about the person's capacity in such circumstances.

Decisions concerning sexual relationships, and the capacity to make these decisions, fall outside the scope of the MCA's framework. However, these decisions do arise frequently in social care contexts, and case law has adopted a slightly different stance to the one codified within the MCA. If the person is unable to (i) describe the nature of the act, (ii) understand the possible consequence of the act including the risk of sexually transmitted diseases, (iii) recognise that the person concerned has a choice and has the right to refuse and (iv) understand the possibility of pregnancy in a heterosexual relationship, then he/she should be considered to lack the capacity to consent (*IM* v. *LM & others* [2014]). This lack of knowledge and understanding may, of course, be due to a lack of education rather than just the person's cognitive impairment. If this is a possibility, the expectation should be that the person would be supported to gain the necessary information. This position also does not mean that responsibility of support staff ends at this point. Continued input and support may still be necessary if the person is identified as being at risk of entering into an abusive and exploitative relationship, regardless of the fact that a determination of capacity has been made.

In social care settings, the notion of a culture change in terms of respect for autonomy is most relevant and has implications for applying the MCA's capacity assessment provisions. Those providing support need to act in a forward-thinking manner that facilitates and involves the person concerned in the day-to-day decisions that they may have to make. This will include the routine support that is offered on a day-to-day basis, but also requires social care staff to be proactive, and to think and plan ahead using more formal tools. With Mrs C, for example, it might well be possible to assist her to make the significant decision about where she receives care, if this is addressed in the early stages of her dementia. This would require advance and personalised care planning, and ensuring that others (including family members) are aware of the relevant supports that need to be put in place to maximise that person's ability to participate in the decision and to exercise a choice. This can be particularly challenging if resources are limited, if there are frequent changes in support staff, or if there are disagreements among family members and others as to what should be done. If the decision that Mrs C needs to make about a care placement is unexpected, then those who know her well will need to ensure that the correct and most relevant information is available and is presented in a way that will optimise her understanding.

Finally, there are also differences in what is expected, depending on the nature, complexity, seriousness and urgency of the decision to be made. The threshold below which someone might be judged on the balance of probabilities to lack capacity should be lower where the outcome is life-determining. In Miss A's situation, for example, support workers will be required to make continuous capacity assessments for each and every decision that they make on behalf of Miss A. These decisions will include what time Miss A gets out of bed, what she eats for breakfast and how she spends her day. Whilst staff should constantly be judging Miss A's decision-making abilities and encouraging her participation in these daily activities, this process will need to be an informal and continuous judgement rather than an explicit and separate process. If not, there is a clear risk that the requirements of providing high-quality care and support to Miss A will be under threat. In contrast, if evidence of her sexual touching of another resident triggers a capacity assessment, the serious question of bodily integrity and sexual freedom will need to be considered carefully, and possibly with additional specialist input from psychiatrists or other suitably experienced professionals.

Determining 'best interests' in social care settings

The MCA also prescribes which approaches to substitute decision-making are lawful for those who lack mental capacity. Of overarching importance in the social care context is the codification of the 'best interests' principle to guide how a decision ought to be made on behalf of an adult who is judged to lack capacity. One immediate difficulty facing all health and other care professionals is that the MCA's approach to best interests aims to shape the process of how to deliberate about the different factors that are relevant to a person's best interests, rather than precisely to determine what best interests actually consists in from a universal legal standpoint (Dunn *et al.*, 2007). There are of course good reasons for this; respect for the person means attending to his/her individual preferences and values in ways that capture a truly person-centred approach to making a judgement about what would be best for him/her. In practice, however, this can raise ethical dilemmas for those who need to apply the law. We consider two types of challenges that can arise.

Balancing past and present wishes, feelings, beliefs and values

It is common for mental incapacity to occur as a result of impairment that arises late in life, after the person has lived a life in which they have developed preferences and values. The ethical principle of respect for precedent autonomy underpins the MCA's framework for substitute decision-making, giving consideration to the person's previous values and preferences, including codifying a role for advance decisions to refuse treatment.

Difficulties can arise, however, when there appears to be direct conflict between these values and the person's in-the-moment preferences. This can be the case for people with dementia, such as Mrs C. If we imagine that Mrs C lacks the capacity to make a decision and it is uncertain whether it would be in her best interests to move her to a care home on the grounds that she had always expressed the view to her children that she never wanted to live in a nursing home, but it was uncertain whether she would actually maintain that view when she moved to the home. If a trial stay at the care home was arranged and Mrs C appeared to really enjoy her new home environment, the challenge in determining her best interests would require her previous values and preferences to be weighed against her current (positive) experiences.

In relation to more day-to-day decisions, a person with dementia who had been a life-long committed vegetarian on moral grounds might find herself distressed when denied the bacon that all other residents were having for breakfast. The relative weights to be given to previous values and current experiences are likely to depend on (i) the strength of the previous values, (ii) what would need to be done to respect these values, (iii) the impact of respecting previous values on current well-being and (iv) the strength of the person's current wishes and desires (Hope *et al.*, 2009).

The best interests of those with life-long, profound intellectual impairments

The focus on determining best interests by reference to a person's past and present wishes, beliefs, feelings and values under the MCA also gives rise to a small but significant group of adults who have life-long and profound disabilities. Those with profound and multiple intellectual disabilities (PMID) are likely to lack, and have lacked, the capacity to make even mundane, everyday decisions for their entire life, and do not offer a clear or interpretable sensory response to any external stimulus. Thus, they have no previous values or wishes on which to base a substitute decision, and it might be challenging or even impossible to ascertain any current experience-driven preferences from them. How should the best interests of these adults be conceptualised?

In practice, there is evidence that support workers in residential care settings draw upon their own life experiences and understanding of a meaningful life in making substitute decisions on behalf of adults with PMID (Dunn *et al.*, 2010). Some have argued for substantive ethical principles such as respect for human dignity to shape decisions in this context (Cantor, 2005), whilst others prefer an approach that recognises, and responds to, the lived realities of people with PMID. This means recognising that people with PMID live alongside other individuals, in families or in communities of residents and caregivers, who do have a range of commitments to comprehensive sets of values, and that drawing on these values, in this context, is a justifiable strategy to adopt (Lim *et al.*, 2016).

Managing the deprivation of a person's liberty

The final component of the MCA's application in social care that we consider is the additional requirements associated with the MCA's Deprivation of Liberty Safeguards (DoLS), introduced in 2007 as part of the legislative process of amending the Mental Health Act 1983. The highly procedural and time- and resource-consuming nature of DoLS has led to questions being raised about their appropriateness. Indeed, the Law Commission has recently recommended their wholesale replacement (Law Commission, 2017), as part of making more general suggestions for improvement to the MCA, and the Government has committed to overhauling and replacing the current DoLS framework with new Liberty Protection Safeguards (LPS), endorsing the Law Commission's recommendations (Department of Health and Social Care, 2018).

The current DoLS review process is undertaken by people specially appointed by the local authority who are required to determine whether, amongst other things, a deprivation of liberty would be in the best interests of the person concerned. DoLS applications and approvals are predominantly made in social care settings; in 2015–2016, over three quarters of all applications came from registered care homes, in both the local authority and private sectors. The key issue for those working in social care is the need to recognise when a deprivation of liberty might be taking place, in order to seek the appropriate authorisations. Following the 2014 Supreme Court judgment in *Cheshire West*, a deprivation of liberty is recognised as having taken place when a person lacks the capacity to consent to care arrangements that involve him/her being subject to continuous supervision or control (for a 'non-negligible period of time'), and where she/he lacks the freedom to leave that continuously supervised or controlling environment. Importantly, whether a deprivation of liberty has occurred is not to be judged by considering the person's degree of impairment or support needs, what a 'normal' life could otherwise be like for that person, or whether she/he is happy and comfortable in the liberty-depriving care setting. This broad and non-relativist account of deprivation of liberty led many care homes to recognise that situations which they thought were merely placing certain restrictions on residents' lives actually qualified as deprivations of liberty, with a ten-fold increase in the number of DoLS applications submitted in England in the year following the *Cheshire West* judgment (Health and Social Care Information Centre, 2015).

For those devising care plans in social care, considering a person's ability to exercise their freedoms within the care environment needs to be foremost in the care planning process. Arrangements that are in the best interests of a person lacking capacity, and that only place restrictions on his/her liberty rather than depriving him/her of his/her liberty, are always to be preferred – and these restrictions should be the least necessary for that person's best interests. Care home staff will need to be imaginative in how they meet the care needs of a person lacking capacity when she/he is behaving in such a way that requires freedom-restricting interventions to be used in the day-to-day delivery of care. After all, care home arrangements can easily slip into DoLS-eligible territory if liberty-restricting steps are imposed for 'non-negligible' periods of time. This might include steps being taken to impose a curfew on a person's movements outside the care home, the use of keypad locks on care home doors to prevent a person from leaving the home without supervision, and instigating a high-degree of observation or control in the home environment itself.

One common issue that can arise in care homes is that a person-centred care decision that triggers a DoLS application for one care home resident might, because of its impact on the entire community of residents, require DoLS applications to be submitted for the other residents. Take the example of a keypad lock on the care home door. If this is introduced to prevent a care home resident who lacks capacity from leaving the home without supervision in his/her best interests, it will likely constitute a deprivation of liberty – particularly if she is only permitted to leave the home on infrequent supervised breaks. However, this lock will have knock-on effects on other residents' freedoms too, which may well not be in these residents' best interests because the lock has not been introduced as a response to their individual needs. Care planning around individual deprivations of liberty must, therefore, take a broad look at any communal 'ripple effects' on the liberty of other residents living in the same environment.

Social care service providers also need to be aware that DoLS applications can only be made from care homes. Other social care services, such as supported living services, shared lives schemes, extra care housing and all forms of domiciliary care fall outside the MCA's DoLS regime. Care arrangements that deprive a person lacking capacity of his/her liberty in his/her best interests in these supported living settings can only be approved by the Court of Protection. It is less likely that deprivations of liberty will arise in such services because care interventions are likely to be less intensive, and the freedom to move around and leave the home environment is widely seen as a defining feature of these care arrangements. However, those working in these supported living services cannot afford to be complacent. Best interests interventions by staff in supported living settings function to (i) restrict the person's ability to access community spaces outside the home, (ii) leave the home, (iii) impose physical restraints on the person or (iv) require very rigid daily regimes to be put in place that might constitute the deprivation of liberty. If so, approval from the Court of Protection will be required. The intention is for the new LPS to apply in all care settings in which the Article 5 right to liberty is engaged (including in domestic settings where the state has positive obligations to meet the care needs of a person lacking capacity).

Conclusion

The MCA has been generally well-received by a social care sector that has long embraced an empowering, person-centred approach to planning and delivering care and support. This partly explains why the MCA has had a positive reception in social care, even if its provisions are not always fully understood or if the lawful basis of substitute decision-making is not explicitly recognised (Manthorpe & Samsi, 2014).

Yet, the close alignment between the ethos of the MCA and social care practice must not function to render invisible certain specific challenges that arise when applying the law in this context. As we have shown in this chapter, such challenges are numerous, and require careful thought in order to be resolved in a legally and ethically sound manner.

First, the assessment of capacity involves specific legal criteria, but it is one that must be situated within interpersonal care relationships and system-level care planning and delivery decisions that must address broader questions of how the needs of social care service users can be best met. Second, the best interests principle needs careful interpretation if it is going to be able to handle wide-ranging decisions from the utterly mundane to the life-changingly important, particularly for adults with dementia and those with learning disabilities whose past and present values, wishes, beliefs and feelings will differ in ethically significant ways. Finally, decisions made on behalf of an individual adult lacking capacity, particularly when these decisions concern the deprivation of his/her liberty, can never be deliberated entirely in isolation from those of other adults who share the communal living environment, and whose own interests and freedoms could negatively be affected by any decisions made. Social care staff need support, resources and experience if they are going to be able to handle the correct application of the MCA in their daily working lives.

References

Cantor, N. (2005) *Making Medical Decisions for the Profoundly Mentally Disabled*. MIT Press.

Department of Health and Social Care (2018) *Final Government Response to the Law Commission's Review of Deprivation of Liberty Safeguards and Mental Capacity: Written statement – HCWS542*. www.parliament.uk/business/publications/written-questions-answers-statements/written-statement/Commons/2018-03-14/HCWS542/.

Dunn, M., Clare, I., Holland, A. & Gunn, M. (2007) Constructing and reconstructing 'best interests': An interpretative examination of substitute decision-making under the Mental Capacity Act 2005. *Journal of Social Welfare and Family Law*, 29, 117–133.

Dunn, M., Clare, I. & Holland, A. (2010) Living 'a life like ours': Support workers' accounts of substitute decision-making in residential care homes for adults with intellectual disabilities. *Journal of Intellectual Disability Research*, 54, 144–160.

Health and Social Care Information Centre. (2015) *Mental Capacity Act 2005, Deprivation of Liberty Safeguards (England) Quarter 4 Return, 2014–15*. https://digital.nhs.uk/data-and-information/publications/statistical/deprivation-of-liberty-safeguards-dols-monthly-summary-statistics/deprivation-of-liberty-safeguards-dols-monthly-summary-statistics-quarter-4-2014-15-january-to-march.

Hope, T., Slowther, A. & Eccles, J. (2009) Best interests, dementia, and the Mental Capacity Act (2005). *Journal of Medical Ethics*, 35, 733–738.

King's Fund (2012) *Demography: Future Trends*. London: King's Fund. www.kingsfund.org.uk/projects/time-think-differently/trends-demography.

Law Commission (2017) *Mental Capacity and Deprivation of Liberty: Report No. 372*. London: Law Commission.

Lim, C. M., Dunn, M. & Chin, J. (2016) Clarifying the best interests standard: The elaborative and enumerative strategies in public policy-making. *Journal of Medical Ethics*, 42, 542–549.

Manthorpe, J. & Samsi, K. (2014) Care homes and the Mental Capacity Act 2005: Changes in understanding and practice over time. *Dementia*, 15, 858–871.

Case law

Airedale NHS Trust v. *Bland* [1993] AC 789.

IM v. *LM & others* [2014] EWCA Civ 37.

LBJ v. *RYJ & VJ* [2010] EWHC 2665.

P v. *Cheshire West, Chester Council and another* [2014] UKSC 19.

Re T (Adult: Refusal of Treatment) [1993] Fam 95.

Re Y (Mental Patient: Bone Marrow Donation) [1997] Fam 110.

Simms v. *Simms and another* [2003] 1 All ER 669.

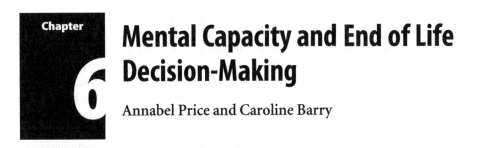

Mental Capacity and End of Life Decision-Making

Annabel Price and Caroline Barry

Impaired capacity towards the end of life is common (Kolva, 2014). Physical frailty, uncontrolled physical symptoms or complications of chronic illness lead to hospital admissions, which are a vulnerable time for those with diminished capacity.

Medically, patients are considered to be approaching end of life if they are likely to die within 12 months (NICE, 2011). Decision-making challenges can arise at any point from diagnosis to death. This chapter outlines some of the common scenarios and dilemmas that can face clinicians, patients and their families during this period. We focus on some of the practical, time-pressured situations likely to arise within the acute hospital, whilst acknowledging the realities of applying the law in an imperfect system. We strive not to provide answers to these difficult questions, but rather to delineate the key points and principles engaged to enable high-quality individualised decision-making.

Diagnosis and treatment

Case study 6.1 Diagnostic uncertainty

A 42-year-old woman with a long history of alcohol excess is admitted to hospital as an emergency with an obstruction of her airway due to a late presentation of a head and neck cancer. She undergoes an emergency tracheostomy which leaves her unable to speak. She appears in shock at her diagnosis and communicates little. The multidisciplinary team attempt to seek her views regarding further treatment for the cancer, but although she is provided with a writing aid she rarely uses this to communicate and when she does write the words are not clear. She is not known to her GP and the social worker in the hospital believes that she may have undiagnosed learning disabilities.

For many people, the diagnosis of a terminal illness is a catastrophic experience. Individuals may use a range of coping mechanisms in order to deal with the existential distress and challenge to personhood a serious illness presents. Mechanisms such as escape-avoidance and distancing are common ways of responding to ill health (Davy, 2000). In addition, difficulties may arise if a patient with impaired capacity is either unable to make a decision, or comes to a treatment decision that clinicians may view as unwise.

The challenge for the clinician when navigating decision-making at this time is differentiating 'normal' illness behaviours (which may influence the patient's ability and willingness to participate in decision-making) from impairment in decision-making function that might engage the diagnostic or functional elements of the Mental Capacity Act 2005 (MCA).

Prevarication over complex decisions is normal. Unfortunately, as described in Chapter 7 [Clinical Ambiguities in the Assessment of Capacity] ambivalence in decision-making may be taken as evidence that a patient lacks capacity to make that decision.

Although the MCA specifically rejects the status approach to capacity, care must be taken to ensure that a causative link is established between diagnostic and functional impairment in capacity (the inability to make the decision is *because of* the dysfunction of mind or brain) in those who find decision-making difficult, before determining that they lack capacity.

In practice, this might mean delaying decisions about proceeding with chemotherapy or surgery until the appropriate level of support is in place (GMC, 2008). This is particularly important following the ruling in *Montgomery* v. *Lanarkshire Health Board* (2015) which confirmed that valid consent relies on the communication of all material risks involved in treatment.

Irrespective of whether the treatment in question is a blood test, or major surgery, there is a statutory presumption in favour of capacity (MCA, Section 1 (2)). This presumption should be exercised in accordance with the civil standard of proof (balance of probabilities) (MCA, Section 2(4)). In the presence of mental illness, presumption of capacity and civil burden of proof may appear an insufficiently robust defence if it allows a patient to refuse life-sustaining treatment, and judicial examination of the facts of a case may yield a different view from the consensus medical opinion.

In the widely reported case of C (*Kings College Hospital NHS Foundation Trust* v. *C & Anor* [2015]), the Court of Protection was asked to consider whether or not a patient had capacity to refuse consent to dialysis following a suicide attempt, in the knowledge that refusal would inevitably result in her death. It was the opinion of two assessing psychiatrists that she lacked capacity to refuse the treatment. Although there was some diagnostic uncertainty, both felt that her presentation was in keeping with a personality disorder, which resulted in an inability to weigh up the information regarding her prognosis.

When deciding the case, MacDonald J found that C was not unable to make a decision regarding renal dialysis. Justifying deviation from the opinion of two experienced psychiatrists as 'a different interpretation of the finely balanced evidence', he acknowledged the benefit provided by 'the entirety of the information available to the court' in coming to his decision. Clinicians must be aware, therefore, that consensus medical opinion from experienced professionals may not always be viewed as the correct 'legal position' when the full facts come before a court, even though the vast majority of medical decisions are decided in this way.

The case of C was notable for clarifying a number of factors concerning decision-making on medical treatment in patients who may have impaired capacity.

First, whilst the MCA is drafted to place the 'diagnostic' test contained in Section 2(1) before the functional test of the capacity assessment in Section 3(1), it is only when a patient is unable to make a decision that the diagnostic element should be considered, and the causative link, if any, between the two tests. The question is not whether the person's ability to make a decision is impaired by the impairment of the mind or brain, but rather whether, on balance of probabilities, they are *unable* to make that decision.

Second, it emphasised that whilst the opinion of clinicians with respect to the diagnosis of an impairment of the mind or brain under Section 2(1) is likely to have determinative weight, the extent to which the diagnosis impairs capacity is ultimately a judicial decision (paragraph 39).

Finally, this case highlights the practical difficulties in respecting a patient's right to come to an 'unwise' decision when it concerns life-sustaining treatment. One particular challenge is assessing capacity in a patient who is categorical and fixed in their decision-making beliefs. It is important not to confuse a capacitous decision to give no weight to important information, such as the likelihood of treatment success, with an inability to use and weigh information in decision-making. In other words:

> a person cannot be considered to be unable to use and weigh information simply on the basis that he or she has applied his or her own values or outlook to that information in making the decision in question and chosen to attach no weight to that information in the decision making process.
>
> [paragraph 38]

Where the patient is unable to give valid consent, clinicians can only provide medical treatment to an individual if it is in their best interests to receive it. In cases of life-prolonging treatment, where the alternative to medical treatment is death, there will be a strong presumption in favour of continuation (MCA Code of Practice).

There are a number of circumstances in which the obligation to provide life-sustaining treatment is displaced. First, by completing a relevant and applicable advance decision to refuse treatment (ADRT). Second, by appointing a lasting power of attorney for welfare, to decline life-sustaining treatment on behalf of the incapacitated person, P (acting in P's best interests according to the MCA). Finally and most commonly, there is no obligation to provide life-sustaining treatment if it is futile or overly burdensome on the individual, and therefore not in P's best interests to receive it (MCA Code of Practice).

When faced with a life-limiting illness, individuals may choose to pursue high-cost, low-evidence-based interventions at personal expense. Such drugs or procedures might not be NHS funded due to high cost or poor evidence base. It is generally accepted that some patients might seek such treatments, even though they are expensive, burdensome and may not bring benefit.

In cases where a person is unable to provide valid consent, many clinicians would struggle to recommend a treatment in the best interests of a vulnerable individual if it involved vast personal expense with no clear benefit. Yet, the courts have confirmed that it may be in the best interests of an individual to receive such treatment if they or their families feel strongly that they want it.

In the case B v. D (2017), the mother of a soldier, D, sought authorisation from the court to allow him to travel abroad for experimental stem cell treatment. That D lacked capacity to consent to this procedure was uncontested. D felt that treatment might improve his brain damage and allow him to be 'normal'. His treating clinicians felt that this would not work and may be harmful. The court found that whilst this might be the case, the psychological impact of being denied the treatment he wanted outweighed the potential harms of the proposed treatment.

One key factor in this case was D's ability to fund his treatment privately. Physicians are ethically and professionally bound to consider the opportunity cost of low benefit interventions. Judges sitting in the Court of Protection are subject to no such restraint, although they cannot mandate that doctors provide treatment to an incapacitated patient that a patient with capacity would not receive (e.g *R(Burke)* v. *General Medical Council* [2005]).

The availability of intensive care beds is one example of day-to day rationing of healthcare resources. It is also an environment where many decisions regarding serious medical treatment are made under the MCA, as the patient is either too unwell, or too sedated, to be able to participate in decision-making.

At the end of life, the benefits and burdens of many interventions become less clear. Up to a third of all patients receive non-beneficial treatment towards the end of life, including intensive care admission, cardiopulmonary resuscitation or chemotherapy (Cardona-Morrell, 2016).

Clinicians may err if they view the benefits and burdens of treatments through a purely medical lens. In *Aintree University Hospital NHS Foundation Trust* v. *James* [2013], the Supreme Court have confirmed that *P*'s best interests must be assessed in a holistic sense, encompassing not just medical factors but the social, psychological and spiritual elements that underpin decision-making.

> The most that can be said, therefore, is that in considering the best interests of this particular patient at this particular time, decision makers must look at his welfare in the widest sense, not just medical but social and psychological; they must consider what the outcome of that treatment for the patient is likely to be; they must try and put themselves in the place of the individual patient and ask what his attitude to the treatment is or would be likely to be; and they must consult others who are looking after him or are interested in his welfare, in particular for their view of what his attitude would be.

Furthermore, whilst the best interests checklist has historically been viewed as non-hierarchical, with all relevant factors being given equal weight, certain factors, such as faith, may attract 'magnetic importance' in decision-making. In practice, this might mean the commencement or continuation of treatments that clinicians feel the patient is unlikely to benefit from.

This has the potential to complicate clinical decision-making, in deciding how much emphasis to place on non-medical factors when determining a patient's best interests. For those who look to the law for clarity, it can seem counterintuitive that there might be more than one 'right' answer to the question: what is in this patient's best interests?

In a recent ethnographic study of conflicts in decision-making trajectories, based in a UK intensive care unit, it was the patients with an uncertain or fluctuating disease trajectory who were most likely to cause conflict or disagreement between clinicians and relatives. Such conflicts were resolved by the removal of medically determined limits of care, such as the rescinding of 'Do Not Resuscitate' [DNACPR] orders or the decision to ventilate a patient when a decision had previously been made not to re-intubate (Higginson *et al.*, 2016).

Evidently, conflict and uncertainty can lead clinicians to change course and provide medical treatments towards the end of life that they might otherwise not. It follows that in determining the best interests of an incapacitated patient, a rigorous examination of all relevant factors should take place before determining the appropriate medical treatment to provide. Whilst analogous to the aims of modern palliative care, to do so may provoke discomfort in many clinicians, who may feel compelled to provide treatment and care that, from a purely medical perspective, is not in that person's best interests.

Hospital admissions and discharges towards the end of life

Case study 6.2 Discharge decision-making

An 88-year-old retired university professor is admitted to hospital due to a care crisis at home. He has lung cancer which has spread to his brain. He has become disinhibited, is impulsive and appears to lack insight into his own physical limitations and his altered personality.

His family are exhausted from a number of disturbed nights, and there is no availability to provide night time care in his area. Despite his wish to be at home, the clinical team and his family feel that his needs would be best met in a setting with 24-hour nursing care.

Discharge planning is a significant issue for acute hospitals, with delayed transfer of care having implications for finance and quality targets. For patients nearing the end of life, delayed discharge may arise due to changes in medical condition, poor communication between departments and difficulties arranging an appropriate care package (Thomas, 2010).

Hospital discharge of the cognitively impaired patient at the end of life has added complexity if it is suspected that they may lack capacity to make an informed decision on place of care on discharge. 'Residence capacity' is a relatively new construct that is gaining increasing prominence in the literature since the MCA came into force.

Effective scrutiny of residence capacity decisions is important, both organisationally in terms of optimising acute bed days and individually in terms of protecting a patient's human rights (Findlay, 2015).

Analysis of personal welfare cases being brought before the Court of Protection demonstrated that questions of care arrangements and residence are a common situation that the court is asked to consider (Series *et al.*, 2017).

Tolerating risky decisions by those with 'borderline' decision-making capacity is likely to present the greatest dilemma; particularly when capacity fluctuates (Brindle, 2004). Decision makers may vary in their interpretation of 'how much' capacity a patient has to demonstrate in order to be judged capacitous.

These cases are a potential source of ethical, in addition to legal, uncertainty. Decision-making involves balancing potentially conflicting values of autonomy, paternalism and resource allocation (Greener, 2012).

When making discharge decisions, clinicians often adopt an 'outcome based' approach; where the perceived need for care home placement drives the capacity and best interests assessment in patients with impaired/borderline capacity. This 'fait a compli' approach to MCA decision-making has been studied by Emmett *et al.* who conducted a large study looking at how judgements about capacity and best interests were made for people with dementia. They found that almost all of the patients they studied who returned to their own home were judged to have capacity and almost all of those who lacked capacity went into care homes. Overcoming the 'protection imperative' that compels clinicians to seek institutionalisation for older, cognitively impaired patients on discharge is challenging even when there is a family carer available to advocate for them (Emmett, 2014).

On the occasions where such cases come before the courts, the judiciary often emphasise the importance of a patient's autonomy, even when they lack capacity to understand the risks of being cared for at home. The prevailing judicial view is provided by the oft-cited Munby J, in the following statement:

Physical health and safety can sometimes be brought at too high a price in happiness and emotional welfare ... what good is it making someone safer if it merely makes them miserable?

(Local Authority X v. MM & Anor [2007])

The elegance of this statement belies the challenges facing decision-making in trying to accommodate those with complex physical and mental needs in the community on discharge. Whilst discharge to a care home may not be the preference of most individuals, the level of care required to support them at home may exceed the financial and/or availability capacity of the organisation(s) responsible for sourcing it.

Provided that the local authority does not act irrationally or unlawfully, it is for them, not judges, to decide how to allocate their budgets (*Westminster City Council* v. *Sykes*). With that in mind, even the most challenging of discharge decisions may be simplified by first establishing what care options are feasible, affordable and available.

Deprivation of Liberty Safeguards

In cases where it is not possible for *P* to consent to their discharge arrangements, clinicians must consider whether it is appropriate to apply the Deprivation of Liberty Safeguards (DoLS).

In theory, DoLS provide statutory means to challenge and scrutinise restrictions placed upon individuals who lack capacity to consent to their care and treatment arrangements. As per chapter 4 (DoLS) clinicians caring for patients who lack capacity are obliged to consider whether the type, nature, duration and intensity of restrictions placed upon incapacitated individuals reach the threshold for a deprivation of liberty. Determining when this threshold is reached can be a challenging task for clinicians caring for patients towards the end of life.

The *Cheshire West* judgment has significantly widened the scope of the safeguards by laying down an 'acid test' of circumstances that are likely to amount to a deprivation of liberty: continuous supervision and control and not free to leave. The care arrangements of those approaching end of life often fulfil the acid test, yet the timescales involved in granting a standard authorisation of a deprivation of liberty commonly exceed the lifespan of the patient, rendering the utility of the exercise questionable.

It is not uncommon for patients within acute hospitals and specialist palliative care units to have care plans which reach the threshold for a deprivation of liberty. Hospices have high staffing ratios, and an acutely unwell patient may have close to one-to-one supervision. Patients who are confused may well have falls-prevention technology, such as bed sensors which prevent them from mobilising without supervision. At the end of life, terminal agitation is very common, often requiring the use of sedation.

The case law surrounding DoLS is complex, ambiguous and at times seemingly contradictory. There is a paucity of case law concerning patients in hospital, and no published judgments considering DoLS in a palliative care setting. Until recently, the decision to apply the DoLS towards the end of life provided an additional administrative burden on staff and an emotional burden on carers due to the mandatory requirement for an inquest.

Whilst the Policing and Crime Act 2017 has removed the need for a mandatory inquest, DoLS remains a poor mechanism to protect the rights of those with impaired capacity towards the end of life.

Those working elsewhere in the acute hospital may find the DoLS less relevant to their practice since the decision in *Ferreira (R (Ferreira)* v. *HM Senior Coroner for Inner South*

London and others [2015]). This case was brought by the relatives of a woman with Down's syndrome who died in intensive care following surgery. The court was asked to consider whether there was a requirement to hold an inquest with a jury, as is required if a person dies in 'state detention'. In the course of the judgment by the Court of Appeal, it was established that the acid test laid down in *Cheshire West* does not extend to the intensive care setting, if the medical treatment in question is indistinguishable to that provided to patients who have capacity to consent to it.

This case was distinguished from *Cheshire West* on the basis that the patient was being treated for a physical illness, and the root cause of her loss of liberty was her physical condition, not any restrictions imposed by the hospital.

Whilst the reasoning behind this judgment at times appears contradictory to the reasoning proposed in *Cheshire West*, this interpretation is now established law following the somewhat surprising decision by a panel of Supreme Court Justices (including, notably, Lady Hale) to refuse permission to appeal.

The impact of this judgment on end-of-life care in other settings is less clear cut. Whilst patients admitted to hospices for end-of-life care may be considered unable to leave because of their physical infirmity, this is not always the case. Often, due to delirium, dementia, brain metastases or medication, a patient may lack insight into their care needs long before their illness renders them immobile. It seems likely that during active treatment, they would be stopped from leaving if a relative tried to remove them, on the grounds that such treatment was in their best interests. Commonly, family members feel unable to meet a patient's care needs at home. Even if *P* feels strongly that they want to be at home, it can be very difficult practically to overcome relatives' objections (Emmett, 2014).

Due to the overwhelming demand placed on local authorities by the *Cheshire West* judgment, many areas are operating a triage system to identify the high-risk cases in which the DoLS are needed most. Those cases in which there is conflict or uncertainty are most likely to attract the attention of managing authorities, if brought to their attention. For the remaining majority of cases, due to the timescales involved, most patients towards the end of life will not have the full benefit of the statutory safeguards the DoLS provide.

The onus remains on healthcare professionals, therefore, to ensure rigorous compliance with all schedules of the MCA DoLS: maximise capacity, minimise restrictions and avoid a deprivation of liberty wherever possible.

Case study 6.3 **Refusing medical treatment**

A 68-year-old retired surgeon with prostate cancer is admitted unwell with renal failure. On admission, he is semi-conscious and unable to consent to treatment. A scan reveals 'back pressure' on the kidneys and an emergency procedure is performed to relieve the obstruction via tubes from the skin to the kidneys (nephrostomy).

Having regained capacity he wants the team to remove the nephrostomies, which he did not consent to, as he would prefer to die peacefully from kidney failure rather than by any other means and wishes to be in control of how he dies.

Wish for hastened death in terminally ill adults

During the passage of the Mental Capacity Bill through Parliament, debate in the House of Lords was dominated by consideration as to whether the Act would provide a vehicle for *'euthanasia by omission'* (Hansard, 2005). Following its assent, the Courts have consistently rejected this interpretation by emphasising that the correct legal starting point is not whether it is lawful to withdraw life-sustaining treatment but rather whether (in persons lacking capacity) it is in that person's best interests to continue to receive it or (if they have capacity) whether they continue to provide valid consent (e.g. *Aintree*).

In recent years, the judiciary have emphasised that the wishes and values of patients must have fundamental importance, irrespective of whether or not a patient has capacity (e.g. *Wye Valley NHS Trust* v. *Mr B* [2015]). In this respect, the MCA mirrors the five priorities for the care of the dying person, which include communicating well and supporting and involving the wishes of the patient in all aspects of their end-of-life care.

A person with capacity may choose to withdraw their consent for life-sustaining medical treatment at any time, even if that decision ultimately results in their death. Clinical guidelines have evolved to reflect this position, for example withdrawal of non-invasive ventilation from patients with motor neurone disease (Association of Palliative Medicine, 2015).

Whilst case law has been clear in establishing the right of the capacitous person to refuse life-sustaining treatment, in some cases such decisions may provoke uncertainty within clinical teams, either because of the 'active' role they may have to play in removing the life-sustaining treatment in question, or because the decision runs against societal norms.

Acquiescing to a request to withdraw medical treatment on which the person is dependent, without due scrutiny of their rationale, although legally sound, could be seen as a failure in the duty of care to patient (e.g. Kerrie Wooltorton) (David *et al.*, 2010).

It may also be relevant to consider the intent of treatment withdrawal: Has the medical treatment become overly burdensome, or is the patient actively attempting to end their life through any available means?

Fleeting thoughts of a wish for hastened death in people nearing the end of life are fairly common whilst more pervasive desire for hastened death is uncommon (Price *et al.*, 2011). Those who have such thoughts however, often fluctuate in their thinking.

Whilst the desire for hastened death is associated with clinical depression (Rayner *et al.*, 2011), the absence of a treatable mental disorder should not exclude exploration of factors which may contribute to the emotional distress such a statement suggests. A stated desire for hastened death may have a range of meanings from an acceptance of impending death to a request for assistance to die (Hudson *et al.*, 2006).

Whether a request for assistance to die is then further considered depends on the legal jurisdiction in which the request is made, and if legal, the conditions under which a request can be met, including whether the person making the request is considered to have mental capacity to make the decision.

Whilst illegal in the UK, physician-assisted suicide has been legalised in a number of jurisdictions in Europe, the USA and in Canada, and is legally permissible in others without statute (e.g. Switzerland). Physician-assisted suicide is the practice of prescribing a lethal dose of medication to a competent person with the intention that the person will take it in order to end their life.

Physician-assisted suicide is usually applicable to people who are terminally ill from a primary physical illness, though in some jurisdictions is available to those with primary psychiatric illness. In European jurisdictions where physician-assisted suicide is illegal, a number of people each year travel to Switzerland and access assisted suicide via organisations such as Exit and Dignitas. In England and Wales, assisting a suicide is punishable by up to 14 years in prison and being in a caring role is a factor in favour of prosecution (CPS, 2010).

In jurisdictions where physician-assisted suicide is legal, competence to make the decision to request assisted suicide is considered an essential safeguard; however, international data on the practice and outcomes of mental capacity assessment for individuals requesting assisted suicide are scarce. There are few mandatory reporting requirements to assess practice and quality of these assessments, even in jurisdictions such as Oregon where annual reports are in the public domain.

Concepts of capacity for assisted suicide vary (Price *et al.*, 2014) and there is little agreement on areas such as what standard of capacity should be met, who is qualified to undertake such assessments or what framework is most appropriate.

The task of capacity assessment becomes even more complex when the request for assisted suicide is driven by suffering due to a primary psychiatric illness that may itself be the main reason why a person's capacity to make decisions may be impaired as well as a key driver for their wish to die (Broome, 2015).

The current lack of clarity needs to be addressed when reviewing existing legislation and considering new legislation (Price, 2015).

Conclusion

In the Courts, best interests decision-making around serious medical treatment is often characterised as a 'matter of life and death' (Baker, 2016). Recent years have demonstrated a clear development in judicial decision-making, where a person's wishes about life-sustaining treatment are increasingly being given much greater weight. Those working within hospitals, however, experience a more nuanced reality. Facilitating 'best interests' decisions in the frail, elderly and incapacitated may be determined by more pragmatic reasoning, such as the availability of care options or a willing family carer. The extent to which a clinical team is willing to tolerate risk, and the weight which they give this is likely to be a key determinant as to whether a patient's wishes are heard and followed. Whilst hospitals and hospices may endeavour to be compliant with deprivation of liberty safeguards, they may find that the practical limitations of applying them limit their usefulness in practice, for the patient and the institution.

The permissibility of medically hastened death for people with life-limiting illness in a growing number of jurisdictions raises clinical, practical and ethical dilemmas for care of patients nearing the end of life. Mental capacity is seen as a key safeguard in any assisted dying legislation but much is unanswered about the effectiveness of this component of the process.

What is clearer is that decision-making at the end of life under the MCA 2005 is no longer a case of 'doctor knows best'. Just as *Montgomery* has rejected the 'responsible body of medical opinion' standard of informed consent, so too has the Court of Protection in determining when it is in the best interests of a patient to withhold or administer life-sustaining treatment, or to decide on their place of care.

It is essential that clinicians place patients at the heart of decision-making and are exhaustive in their attempts to determine what their past and present wishes and values are. Whilst there is always the option to seek clarification from the courts, the emotional and financial costs, even in undisputed cases, should not be underestimated.

These authors would argue that supported decision-making is the keystone of good clinical practice and, wherever possible, should remain at the bedside.

References

Association of Palliative Medicine (2015)
Withdrawal of Assisted Ventilation at the
Request of a Patient with Motor Neurone
Disease. Guidance for Professionals. APM.

Baker, J. (2014) A matter of life and death.
Oxford Shrieval Lecture 11 October 2016.
www.judiciary.gov.uk/wp-content/uploads/
2016/10/mr-justice-baker-shrieval-lecture-
11102016.pdf.

Brindle, N. & Holmes, J. (2004) Capacity and
coercion: Dilemmas in the discharge of older
people with dementia from general hospital
settings. *Age and Ageing*, 1, 16–20.

Broome, M. R. & de Cates, A. (2015) Choosing
death in depression: A commentary on
'Treatment-resistant major depressive
disorder and assisted dying'. *Journal of
Medical Ethics*, 41(8), 586–587.

Cardona-Morrell, M., Kim, J. C. H., Turner, R.
M., Anstey, M., Mitchell, I. A. & Killman, K.
(2016) Non-beneficial treatments in hospital
at the end of life: A systematic review on the
extent of the problem. *International Journal
for Quality in Health Care*, 28(4), 456–469.

Crown Prosecution Service (2010) Assisted
suicide policy. www.cps.gov.uk/publications/
prosecution/assisted_suicide_policy.html.

Davy, J. & Ellis, S. (2000) *Counselling Skills in
Palliative Care*. Open University Press.

Department for Constitutional Affairs (2007)
Mental Capacity Act 2005: Code of Practice.
London: HMSO.

David, A. S., Hotopf, M., Moran, P., Owen, G.,
Szmukler, G. et al. (2010) Mentally
disordered or lacking capacity? Lessons for
management of serious deliberate self harm.
British Medical Journal, 341, c4489.

Emmett, C., Poole, M., Bond, J. & Hughes, J.
(2014) A relative safeguard? The informal
roles that families and carers play when
patients with dementia are discharged from
hospital into care in England and Wales.
*International Journal of Law, Policy and
Family*, 28(3), 302–320.

Findlay, D. (2015) But when can I go home?
Commentary on . . . residence capacity.
British Journal of Psychiatry Advances, 2(52),
313–314.

General Medical Council (2008) *Consent:
Patients and doctors making decisions
together*. GMC Hansard.

Greener, H., Poole, M., Emmett, C., Bond, J.,
Louw, S. & Hughes, J. (2012) Value
judgement and conceptual tension: Decision-
making in relation to hospital discharge for
people with dementia. *Clinical Ethics*, 7(4),
166–174.

Higginson, I., Rumble, C., Shipman, C., et al.
(2016) The value of uncertainty in critical
illness? An ethnographic study of patterns
and conflicts in care and decision making
trajectories. *BMC Anaesthesiology*, 16, 11.

Hudson, P., Kristjanson, L. J., Ashby, M., Kelly,
B., Schofield, P., Hudson, R. et al., (2006)
Desire for hastened death in patients with
advanced disease and the evidence base of
clinical guidelines: A systematic review.
Palliative Medicine, 20(7), 693–701.

Leadership Alliance for the Care of Dying
People (2014) *One Chance to Get It Right*.
London: HMSO.

Kolva, E., Rosenfield, B., Brescia, R. & Comfort,
C. (2014) Assessing decision-making capacity
at the end of life. *General Hospital Psychiatry*,
36, 392–397.

Mackenzie, J., Lincoln, N. & Newby, G. (2008)
Capacity to make a decision about
discharge destination after a stroke: A pilot
study. *Clinical Rehabilitation*, 22(12),
1116–1126.

National Institute for Health and Care
Excellence (2011) *Quality Standard 13 End of
Life Care for Adults*. NICE.

Price, A. (2015) Mental capacity as a safeguard
in assisted dying: Clarity is needed. *BMJ*, 351,
h4461.

Price, A., McCormack, R., Wiseman, T. &
Hotopf, M. (2014) Concepts of mental
capacity for patients requesting assisted
suicide: A qualitative analysis of expert
evidence presented to the Commission on
Assisted Dying. *BMC Medical Ethics*, 15, 32.

Price, A., Lee, W., Goodwin, l., Rayner, L.,
Humphreys, R., Hansford, P., Sykes, N.,
Monroe, B., Higginson, I. J. & Hotopf, M.
(2011) Desire for death in a palliative
population. *BMJ Supportive and Palliative
Care*, 1, 140–148.

Rayner, L., Lee, W., Price, A., Monroe, B., Sykes, N., Hansford, P., Higginson, I. J. & Hotopf, M. (2011) The clinical epidemiology of depression in palliative care and the predicative value of somatic symptoms: Cross survey and four week follow up. *Palliative Medicine*, 25(3), 229–241

Series, L., Fennell, P., Doughty, J. & Mercer, A. (2017) *Welfare Cases in the Court of Protection: A Statistical Overview*. Nuffield Foundation.

Thomas, C. & Ramcharan, A. (2010) Why do patients with complex palliative care needs experience a delayed hospital discharge? *Nursing Times*, 106(25), 15–17.

Case law

Aintree University Hospitals NHS Foundation Trust v. *James* [2013] UKSC 67.

B v. *D* [2017] EWCOP 15.

C (Kings College Hospital NHS Foundation Trust) v. *C & Anor* [2015] EWCOP 80.

Cheshire West and Chester Council v. *P* [2014] UKSC 19.

HM Coroner – Great Norfolk District, Kerrie Wooltorton Inquest (2009).

Local Authority X v. *MM & Anor* [2007] EWHC 2689.

Montgomery v. *Lanarkshire Health Board* [2015] UKSC 11.

R (Burke) v. *General Medical Council* [2005] EWCA Civ 1003.

R (Ferreira) v. *HM Senior Coroner for Inner South London* [2015] EWHC 2990.

Westminster City Council v. *Sykes* [2014] EWCOP B9.

Wye Valley NHS Trust v. *Mr B* [2015] EWCOP 60.

Clinical Ambiguities in the Assessment of Capacity

Elizabeth Fistein and Rebecca Jacob

Medical practitioners have long voiced their frustrations about the development of legal tests that are difficult to apply to clinical situations, as exemplified by this quote from Roth *et al.* (1977):

> The search for a single test of competency is a search for a Holy Grail. In practice, judgements of competency go beyond semantics or straightforward applications of legal rules; such judgements reflect social considerations and societal biases as much as they reflect matters of law and medicine.

Even when the legal test itself is clear and simple, the process of applying it to the complex situations that arise in clinical medicine is not. This problem was recognised by Dame Elizabeth Butler-Sloss:

> The general law on mental capacity is, in my judgment, clear and easily to be understood by lawyers. Its application to individual cases in the context of a general practitioners surgery, a hospital ward and especially in an intensive care unit is infinitely more difficult to achieve
>
> (*Re B*, 2002).

Legislation pertaining to health, social care and financial decisions on behalf of those with impaired decision-making capacity (DMC) came into being with the introduction of the Mental Capacity Act (MCA) 2005. The Code of Practice, published soon after, appears to give clear and concise guidance on the treatment of people with impaired DMC (MCA Code of Practice, 2007). However, despite this seemingly explicit guidance, the application of the law in clinical settings is far from straightforward (Herring, 2008).

This may be related to the following observations:

- The law imposes a dichotomy (competent v. incompetent) on what is arguably a spectrum of ability, with most people having some degree of DMC.
- The law focuses on cognitive abilities (to understand, retain and use information relevant to the decision), whereas in practice many difficulties appear to be related to a patient's emotional ambivalence regarding their decision.
- The law acknowledges that DMC may fluctuate but in practice it may be difficult to determine when to intervene.
- The law is clear that people have the right to make a decision for any reason, or no reason at all, but in practice it can be difficult to decide how much weight to give to unusual beliefs which could impair the ability to evaluate relevant information.
- The law defines DMC as decision specific, but in practice there is a risk of unwittingly adopting a status- or diagnosis-based approach to determining DMC in particular patient groups.

Decision-making capacity: a spectrum of ability with a legal threshold

As described in earlier chapters, the functional approach (Grisso *et al.*, 1997) has now been accepted in many jurisdictions as the most appropriate legal test of DMC. Its use has replaced the status approach, which relies on a person's condition or diagnosis as a marker of competence, and the outcome approach, which focuses on whether or not a patient's decision appears 'sound or reasonable'. The Mental Capacity Act 2005 creates a statutory duty to perform a functional assessment of DMC, or the ability to make a particular decision at a particular time, which seems at first to be both clear and precise.

However, in some respects, DMC lies on a dimensional scale and its determination is not always a simple black and white issue. As Thorpe J comments in his ruling in *Re C*:

> If the patient's capacity to decide is unimpaired, autonomy weighs heavier but the further capacity is reduced, the lighter autonomy weighs.
>
> (*Re C*, 1994)

The fact that an individual's DMC can be 'reduced' suggests that it is not, in fact, an all or nothing ability. It is the law that imposes a dichotomy (competent v. incompetent) on what is arguably a spectrum of ability. There is an expectation that, concerning a specific question and at a specific time, an individual either does or does not have legal capacity to make his or her own decision. Whether or not he or she has reached this point where his or her ability to make this particular decision is so impaired that he or she should be judged unable to decide is a matter of judgement. This lack of certainty, and the requirement to make a binary decision based on an ability usually better understood as moving along a sliding scale, may feel unsatisfactory when treating a patient against his or her wishes.

How then should clinicians approach cases where the legal test of capacity is difficult to apply? Ideally, legal advice must be easily accessible for cases that appear controversial because of the issues relating to the assessment of DMC. The following examples, drawn from case law, typify some of the contentious issues faced by clinicians. The problems considered are: how to respond when the patient seems ambivalent about his or her own decision; when to intervene in cases of fluctuating capacity; how much weight to give to unusual beliefs; how to avoid unwittingly adopting a status-based approach to capacity in particular patient groups. They are discussed in some detail, in order to illustrate the current legal position and to provide some guidance for clinicians who may encounter similar cases. Finally, the management of self-harm, a situation that often raises all of the issues discussed in this chapter, is reviewed and relevant cases are discussed.

Ambivalence

Assessing the capacity of people who are ambivalent about treatment can be particularly complex. Ambivalence in this context implies that an individual has difficulties in coming to a decision about the treatment in question and vacillates between accepting or refusing treatment. This may suggest that the person is experiencing difficulty with the third component of the capacity test laid down in the MCA 2005: that he or she is unable to use or weigh information relevant to the decision. Alternatively, it may simply indicate that the decision to be made is difficult or finely balanced and that therefore a degree of vacillation might be expected.

The issue of apparent ambivalence was considered by the courts prior to the introduction of the MCA 2005.

> Ms B, a 43-year-old woman who was paralysed from the neck down and dependent on artificial ventilation refused this intervention shortly after it was introduced despite being made aware that ventilatory support was necessary to preserve life.
>
> (Re B, 2002)

The doctors used the argument that they could not take her decision to discontinue treatment as final because she vacillated in her decision-making process. It is clear that the greater the vacillation in decision-making, the more likely it is that an individual will be regarded as unable to make their own decision.

Is ambivalence per se a sign of impaired DMC? There is, after all, an expectation that, if capable, the individual should come to some conclusion regarding treatment. However, when should a decision be accepted as final? The danger is that health professionals may accept the decision that they consider reasonable, even if the patient continues to vacillate. Yet another question arises: should a refusal of life-preserving treatment be automatically suspect? And, given the irreversible consequences of such a decision, how long should a health professional wait for a possible change of heart before the decision is accepted?

Starting from the presumption that all adults possess capacity unless proven otherwise, Dame Butler-Sloss found that Ms B was indeed competent to refuse ventilation, stressing the duty to respect competent patients' refusals of treatment, and the right of patients to change their minds:

> I am entirely satisfied that Ms. B is competent to make all relevant decisions about her medical treatment including the decision whether to seek to withdraw from artificial ventilation. Her mental competence is commensurate with the gravity of the decision she may wish to make.
> I would like to add how impressed I am with her as a person, with the greatest courage, strength of will and determination she has shown in the last year, with her sense of humour, and her understanding of the dilemma she has posed to the hospital. She is clearly a splendid person and it is tragic that someone of her ability has been struck down so cruelly. I hope she will forgive me for saying, diffidently, that if she did reconsider her decision, she would have a lot to offer the community at large.

It would seem erroneous on reflection to assume that some ambivalence when faced with life-preserving healthcare decisions is abnormal or, to use the wording of the MCA 2005, indicative of 'an impairment of, or a disturbance in the *functioning* of, the *mind* or *brain*'. A more complex procedure would require a greater commitment from the patient when consenting and may have more profound health consequences. Accordingly, it would stand to reason that a level of uncertainty, fear and vacillation could be evident and clinicians must take this into account when making assessments of decision-making capacity. In other words, ambivalence should not be assumed equivalent to incapacity. The test is whether or not the patient, as a result of disorder or dysfunction of brain or mind, is *unable* to weigh the information relevant to the decision. The fact that a decision is a difficult one, with irreversible consequences requiring careful consideration, must not, in itself, be taken to mean that the person, who is in the unfortunate position of having to make that decision, lacks capacity (Gunn, 1994).

The process of assessing capacity in the face of ambivalence becomes more complicated when the person in question is affected by a relapsing and remitting mental illness, as in the 2013 Court of Protection case *Re SB (A Patient: Capacity to Consent to Termination)*.

SB, a 37-year-old graduate and IT professional, had an eight-year history of bipolar affective disorder but did not accept that she had a mental illness and had, at various times, been detained for compulsory psychiatric treatment. Two years prior to the case, she had experienced an unplanned pregnancy in the early stages of a new relationship, and had taken the decision to undergo termination of the pregnancy by medical induction of labour at 19 weeks as she was concerned about the potential teratogenic effects of her psychiatric medication. She subsequently married her partner, decided that she would like to have a baby (although her husband was not so enthusiastic), conceived and was 23 weeks pregnant at the time of the case.

In his judgment, Holman J noted that for the first 17–18 weeks of the pregnancy she 'showed every sign of wanting to keep this baby and of desiring to be a loving and caring mother to the baby'. She then discontinued her psychiatric medication and appeared to relapse, allegedly becoming physically aggressive towards her husband. Her attitude towards her pregnancy also changed completely, and she attended a clinic, seeking a termination. An appointment was made for a surgical termination, but she did not attend, later stating that this was because she would have preferred to undergo a medical induction of labour, as she had done for her previous termination. Shortly after this, she was detained under the Mental Health Act. She continued to maintain that she wished to have a termination of pregnancy but her psychiatrist judged her to lack the necessary DMC to consent to the procedure. Expert psychiatric evidence stated that, whilst SB 'perfectly' understood what was involved in a termination, and the irreversible consequences of the procedure, she was 'only making this decision to seek a termination because of the skewed thought processes and paranoid beliefs as a result of her illness … it therefore follows that she lacks capacity to make this important decision'. SB's psychiatrists were concerned that, because of her illness, she was unable to understand, use or weigh the information that, contrary to her beliefs since relapsing, her husband and mother were caring and supportive, and would help her to look after the baby if she decided to carry the pregnancy to term. In their opinion, this information was relevant to SB's decision.

Holman J did not accept this conclusion, stating that:

What weighs most significantly with me is that, even if the patient has some skewed thoughts and paranoid or delusional views with regard to her husband and his attitude towards her and his behaviour, she gives many other reasons for desiring a termination.

He accepted that it was possible that, as SB stated, the state of her relationship with her husband had deteriorated since she became pregnant. He also stated that, even if SB was mistaken about the commitment of her husband to her, it was undoubtedly the case that she had now been detained under the Mental Health Act and that she felt unable to continue a pregnancy under those circumstances.

Despite the 'strong temporal relationship between the patient stopping medication, developing paranoid ideas about her husband or mother and deciding to opt for a termination of her pregnancy' her decision was based on other reasons, and she retained the ability to understand, retain, weigh up and use the information relating to those reasons. Her change of heart about the pregnancy was not, therefore, evidence of a loss of DMC but, at least in part, a response to a change in her personal circumstances (*Re SB (A Patient: Capacity to Consent to Termination)*).

- A person with legal capacity may consent to treatment and later refuse it (or vice versa) without ever having impaired DMC. Both decisions are valid and should be respected – patients have the right to change their minds.
- A person with impaired DMC may also consent to treatment and later refuse it (or vice versa) without ever regaining legal capacity. A change of heart leading to assent to the course of action recommended by healthcare professionals should not, in itself, be taken as evidence of restoration of legal capacity and best interests principles will still apply

Fluctuating capacity

Another difficulty arises in cases of fluctuating DMC. The ability to make a particular decision at a specific time may be based on a number of factors, including physical health, intoxication with substances and mental state, meaning someone may be able to make a decision at one time but be incapable of making the same decision at another time. When an individual is deemed to lack legal capacity, a judgment must be made as to whether treatment can be delayed until the patient's DMC improves sufficiently for them to make the decision. An example of this is alcohol intoxication, which is a common complicating factor when treatment decisions need to be made for patients who self-harm (Hawton *et al.*, 1989). The difficulty is in deciding whether to treat immediately, in the patient's best interests, or whether it would be reasonable to wait till they are sober and seek their consent to the necessary treatments. The pivotal deciding factor in these cases appears to be whether the situation is an emergency or not, a clinical rather than a legal decision.

Prior to the MCA 2005, fluctuating DMC could lead to a finding that the patient lacked legal capacity. The case of *Re R* (1991) illustrates this point.

R, a 15-year-old girl who was suffering from severe mental health problems, refused the administration of anti-psychotic drugs. Her capacity was questioned due to the fact that on occasion she did not appear able to make a fully informed refusal of treatment, although at other times she did appear more lucid and able to make a choice.

Lord Donaldson stated that it was clearly in *R*'s best interests to have treatment and, as she was not in a position to give a competent decision due to her fluctuating DMC, the decision was taken out of her hands and she was given the necessary treatment.

However, under the Mental Capacity Act 2005, fluctuating DMC is by no means considered equivalent to legal incapacity. Section 4(3) states that, when determining the best interests of a person with impaired DMC who currently cannot make a decision, you 'must consider (a) whether it is likely that the person will at some time have capacity in relation to the matter in question, and (b) if it appears likely that he will, when that is likely to be'. Section 4(4) continues that you 'must, so far as reasonably practicable, permit and encourage the person to participate, or to improve his ability to participate, as fully as possible in any act done for him and any decision affecting him'. These clauses are consistent with the second of the five principles on which the MCA is based: 'A person is not to be treated as unable to make a decision unless all practicable steps to help him to do so have been taken without success.'

The duty to maximise capacity requires us to delay the decision, whenever possible, to allow the patient to decide during a period of lucidity. During such an interval, the patient can make contemporaneous decisions about immediate treatment, make an Advance Decision to Refuse Treatment, nominate someone to make decisions about their best interests using a lasting power of attorney, and give a clear statement of wishes and preferences that can be used as the basis for best interests decision-making, should this become necessary in the future. (It must also be noted that, in the case of a mentally ill patient detained under the Mental Health Act (MHA) 1983, an advance decision to refuse medical treatment for mental disorder may be overridden.)

If treatment is needed during a period of incapacity and it is not clinically acceptable to wait for a potential lucid period, best interests principles apply. The treating clinician must make the choice as to the best interests of the patient after ascertaining from relatives, or an independent mental capacity advocate, the previously expressed wishes of the patient (MCA Code of Practice, 2007). This will involve careful consideration of views expressed by the patient during periods of lucidity. Dame Butler-Sloss describes patients' best interests as determined by taking 'into account a wide range of ethical, social, moral, emotional and welfare considerations' (Re B, 2002), suggesting this encompasses far more than merely the treatment decision at hand. In 2012, the Court of Protection considered a case which, amongst other things, concerned the duty to try to restore capacity: A Local Authority v. E (by her Litigation Friend the Official Solicitor) [2012] EWHC 1639 (COP).

E, a 32-year-old former medical student, had suffered from extremely severe anorexia nervosa since the age of 11. Although she had shown a positive response to treatment when younger, for the six years preceding the case she remained extremely unwell, spending long periods of time in hospital without experiencing any sustained benefit from the treatment provided. In 2011, she signed an advance decision to refuse medical treatment, with a view to preventing others from feeding her. Two periods of treatment under the Mental Health Act followed, but no sustained improvement resulted. The team treating her reached the conclusion that it was no longer appropriate to use the MHA to enforce treatment, and E was admitted to a community hospital for palliative care, on an 'end-of-life' pathway with high doses of opiate medication. A declaration was sought from the Court of Protection that this course of action was lawful.

Mr Justice Peter Jackson applied the MCA in order to reach a decision. On the basis of expert evidence, he identified two possible courses of action: to continue with palliative care, which would result in E dying in the near future, or admitting E to a specialist unit for tube-feeding under sedation in intensive care for a period of a year or more, a treatment plan which might return E to 'relatively normal life' and had not yet been tried. This second course of action was, apparently, prevented by the Advance Decision to Refuse Treatment which E had signed in 2011. Jackson J noted that, at the time E made the advance decision to refuse tube-feeding, her BMI was very low (briefly peaking at 15), and that 'her obsessive fear of weight gain makes her incapable of weighing the advantages and disadvantages of eating in any meaningful way. For *E*, the compulsion to prevent calories entering her system has become the card that trumps all others'. He concluded that the advance decision was not valid, as *E* had not had the necessary DMC at the time she made it, and that she continued to lack legal capacity to make decisions about her treatment, particularly as she was, by the time the case came to court 'subject to strong sedative medication and ... in a severely weakened condition'.

Furthermore, he noted the hope that 'with refeeding, *E* will reach the point where her weight stabilises at a more normal level (in the order of BMI 17) and leads her to recover the capacity to take decisions for herself'. This was not a course of action without risks – insertion of a PEG tube alone carried an immediate 2–3% mortality risk, and likelihood of recovery was estimated to be around 20%. However, Jackson J ruled that this option should be taken, as it was in *E*'s best interests to try to restore her health and her capacity, at least enough for her to make the decision about further treatment for herself:

> For present purposes, I find nothing in *E*'s statements to indicate a belief that, if she were well, she would not want efforts to be made to save her. Although the risks of treatment are high and the chances of recovery are low, these are odds that patients and doctors (and *E* would by now be a doctor but for her illness) willingly accept when considering life-saving medical treatment in other circumstances.

- In cases of fluctuating DMC, if treatment is needed during a period of incapacity and it is not clinically acceptable to wait for a potential lucid period, best interests principles apply.
- An Advance Decision to Refuse Treatment is only valid if the person making it has the legal capacity at the time.

Unusual values/belief systems

A further area of complexity is the relevance of values or belief systems that may influence an individual's decision-making capacity. There is an understanding, shaped by case law, that a decision which might be influenced by a set of values or religious beliefs should be respected. The example of a Jehovah's Witness refusing to accept a blood transfusion on the grounds of his or her religious beliefs is often used to illustrate this point. Without background knowledge of the dogma on which this belief system is centred, such a stance might make one question the patient's mental state and suspect a mental disorder.

However, what about more idiosyncratic beliefs that may indicate the presence of a mental disorder? Psychiatric delusions, particularly of persecution, might make a patient believe wrongly that a treatment will do him harm rather than good. Alternatively a patient with a psychotic depression might have delusions of guilt or worthlessness (Carpenter *et al.*, 2000), she might be convinced that she deserves the illness and is not worthy of help. In some cases, it might be appropriate to use the Mental Health Act 1983, to provide treatment for the underlying mental disorder. However, not all mentally ill people meet criteria for compulsory treatment under the MHA, which states that the patient must have a mental disorder of a nature and degree that requires hospital treatment, and that this is the least restrictive treatment option. Furthermore, the MHA does not provide any legal justification for the provision of treatment for physical conditions in the absence of consent. If such treatment were required, it would be important to make an assessment of whether the delusions impact on a patient's decision-making capacity as defined by the MCA. In particular, delusions or cognitive bias arising as a result of serious mental illness may render a patient unable to give appropriate weight to relevant information and so come to a decision.

When a belief system is shared by a group of individuals, it is easier to accept and understand how it might influence decision-making. The problem that confounds clinicians is when and under what circumstances should we treat an individual's belief system as reason for questioning their capacity to make decisions? This inevitably becomes relevant in the context of a refusal of treatment. As outlined in earlier chapters, the MCA imposes a presumption of capacity for all adults. Findings of incapacity can only be made in the context of 'an impairment of, or a disturbance in the functioning of, the mind or brain'. When applying the MCA, unless there is an identifiable mental disorder, value systems must be accepted.

The case of *Re SB*, introduced earlier in this chapter, illustrates the difficulty of applying the legal test of capacity in the context of psychotic illness. It appears likely that, upon experiencing a relapse in her bipolar affective disorder, *SB*'s attitude towards her husband and her mother had changed quite dramatically, to the extent that she had been physically violent towards her husband, and believed that he and her mother, who were both expressing their willingness to support her with pregnancy and parenthood, were not actually supportive of her. At the same time, she sought termination of a pregnancy that she had previously shown every sign of wishing to carry to term. This raised a number of difficult questions for the treating team and the court: was *SB*'s belief that her family were rejecting her based in reality or was it delusional, and, if her belief was delusional, was it relevant to her decision to seek a termination? Only if her beliefs were pathological, and her decision to seek a termination rested on the presence, or absence, of family support, could *SB* be found to lack the DMC to make her own decision to have a termination. Furthermore, her history of undergoing termination of a previous pregnancy suggests that this was not a procedure that was in conflict with *SB*'s underlying value system.

Even more difficult than cases of relapsing and remitting illness are cases of chronic mental ill-health, where the distinction between beliefs induced by illness and long-standing fundamental values becomes blurred. As Jackson J put it in the case of *E* (described earlier in this chapter):

> The beliefs and values that would be likely to influence *E*'s decision if she had capacity are not easy to articulate. It depends upon an assessment of her true identity. Has she been so ill for so long that her illness would remain part of who she is, even if she had capacity? Or is she still the person she was before anorexia took her in its grip? Looking ahead, will *E* always see herself as a victim, or can she come to see herself as a survivor? In the end, only *E* can know the answers to these questions.

- Unusual beliefs in the absence of 'an impairment of, or a disturbance in the functioning of, the mind or brain' cannot be interpreted as evidence of impaired DMC.
- In the context of mental ill-health, unusual beliefs can only be considered to impair DMC if they lead to a decision that the person would not have made had they not been unwell.

Incapacity in vulnerable populations

There is now a substantial empirical literature about the DMC of different groups of adults, including those with physical illness, mental illness, dementia and intellectual disabilities.

Generally, but by no means inevitably, people with mental disorders, particularly psychosis, are more likely than their 'general population' counterparts to experience impairments in their DMC (Wong *et al.*, 1999, Bellhouse *et al.*, 2003, Owen *et al.*, 2009). However, this does not mean that legal incapacity can be presumed on the basis of the presence of a particular type of behaviour, symptom or diagnosis.

Consider the following incorrect assumptions which could be made in response to the cases outlined in this chapter.

- Re B – a decision to refuse life-sustaining treatment must be evidence of mental ill-health.
- Re SB – a change of heart occurring during an episode of mental ill-health must be evidence of loss of DMC.
- Re R – fluctuating capacity must mean that the patient is incapable of making the decision themselves.
- Re SB – a decision made at a similar time to the development of delusional beliefs must have been made because of the delusional beliefs.

Research has suggested that those conditions affecting insight, or understanding of the illness, are more likely than other forms of mental ill-health to impair DMC. Psychotic disorders are characterised by their likelihood to distort reality and a lack of acceptance of illness and therefore this encroaches onto patients' understanding of the existence of illness and the need for treatment. Conditions like depression, however, are less likely to distort understanding although depression and psychosis are not mutually exclusive conditions (Grisso *et al.*, 1991, 1995).

Furthermore, a number of studies have suggested that impaired DMC is commonly seen amongst patients suffering with neurological disorders, including dementia and learning disabilities (Marson *et al.*, 1996). Studies have also found impaired DMC in people with a variety of medical disorders, usually those affecting the higher cognitive functions (Raymont *et al.*, 2004). Intuitively, this is what one would expect, as the functional assessment of capacity does require cognitive abilities related to reasoning, understanding, memory and executive function.

- Mental illness, especially where insight is impaired, may impact upon DMC.
- However, many people experiencing mental illness retain the DMC necessary to make their own decisions about treatment, and physical illness can also impair DMC.
- Decisions concerning legal capacity to make treatment decisions must be based upon a functional assessment of ability to understand, retain, use and weigh the information relevant to the decision, and not based on assumptions arising from a particular diagnosis or symptom.

Self-harm and consent/refusal of treatment

A not-infrequent contentious issue in clinical practice is the treatment of individuals who self-harm. Self-harm has been variously defined and, over the years, the terms deliberate self-harm, intentional self-harm, parasuicide, attempted suicide, non-fatal suicidal behaviour and self-inflicted violence have all been used to describe the act. More recently, the National Institute of Clinical Excellence (NICE) have suggested the use of the term 'self-harm', which patients seem to find more acceptable and less pejorative. NICE have defined self-harm, in their guidelines pertaining to the management of self-harm, as: Self-poisoning or self-injury, irrespective of the apparent purpose of the act (NICE, 2004).

Self-harm is seen frequently within emergency medical practice, and can prove challenging for physicians and psychiatrists. Managing a case of self-harm will sometimes raise all of the issues discussed so far in this chapter – ambivalence, fluctuating capacity, unusual values – and the treatment of vulnerable groups who are prone to be labelled as lacking the capacity to make their own decisions.

Self-harm is a complex behaviour that can best be thought of as a maladaptive response to acute and chronic stress, often but not exclusively linked with thoughts of suicide. Many of those who harm themselves may have a severe mental disorder and/or have misused alcohol; it is not uncommon for people who have deliberately harmed themselves to refuse treatment, despite attending the A&E department seemingly of their own free will (Hassan et al., 1999, Jacob et al., 2005).

This pattern of attending hospital but refusing treatment may seem surprising or contradictory. Treatment refusal may be understood in the context of suicidal intent, which not uncommonly triggers self-harm. However, many acts of self-harm are not directly associated with suicidal intent. They are often an attempt to communicate with others, to secure help, or to obtain relief from a difficult and otherwise overwhelming situation or emotional state. The fact that people attend hospital at all may signal their degree of uncertainty or ambivalence about their intended actions. When viewed in the context of complex mental processes, the behaviour is more easily understood, but in the setting of a busy A&E department, the management of these patients is particularly challenging. It is important to adopt an empathic, non-judgemental approach and to avoid the 'malignant alienation' that can increase risk of subsequent suicide (Mackay et al., 2005).

Irrespective of the events leading to an admission to an A&E department, it remains the duty of the treating team to assess an individual's capacity when dealing with refusal of treatment. This process can be pivotal in resolving the conflict, which arises between respect for autonomy and an individual's need for care and protection from harm. People who have recently harmed themselves often have fluctuating capacity due to the physical effects of their act of self-harm or the misuse of alcohol. There is sometimes confusion amongst healthcare professionals regarding the management of patients who refuse treatment, due to the law's disparate treatment of those with mental illness and those with physical illness (Szmukler, 2004). On the face of it, those with physical health needs, such as suturing, surgery or the administration of an antidote to self-poisoning, must give consent before such a procedure is carried out, and the refusals of those who have capacity must be respected, although those who lack capacity must still be given emergency treatment if it is judged necessary to the best interests of the patient.

This was the difficulty faced by the emergency department team involved in the case of Kerrie Wooltorton, a young woman who developed renal failure following the deliberate consumption of anti-freeze. She had called an ambulance so that she could end her life without discomfort in hospital, rather than alone at home. She refused all active treatment proposed to save her life, and produced a written statement, which made it clear that she wished to refuse treatment even though her death would be the likely consequence. The treating team judged that Ms Wooltorton retained the capacity to make her own decision about treatment and that they could not, therefore, impose treatment to save her life in the absence of her consent.

The reports of this case in the media understandably raised questions and concerns amongst physicians and psychiatrists alike (David *et al.*, 2010, Mclean, 2009). In response, Professor Louis Appleby, the National Director for Mental Health, sought to clarify the legal duties and powers of doctors in an open letter to the Royal College of Psychiatrists (2009) in which he stated:

> On the general issue, there are two key points that I would make. The first is that it has been established (e.g. by the case of *B* v. *Croydon Health Authority*) that treatment for mental disorder under the Mental Health Act can include treatment of the physical consequences of self-harm, which results from that disorder ... The second point is that it is possible for someone to meet the criteria for detention under the [Mental Health] Act even though they retain the capacity to take decisions about their treatment.

So, as discussed above, competent refusals to accept physical treatment for a mental disorder may sometimes be overridden, using the Mental Health Act 1983. The Mental Health Act is concerned with a patient's health and safety and also the risk of others, therefore when a section for assessment or treatment is considered, the best interests of more than just the patient are considered. Certain cases have suggested that self-harm may be a behavioural extension of an underlying mental illness and should therefore be treated, if the criteria are met, under the aegis of the Mental Health Act 1983, even where treatment is refused. The leading case, mentioned by Professor Appleby in his letter on the Wooltorton Case, is that of *B* v. *Croydon Health Authority* (1995) in which the Court of Appeal reviewed the substantive issues relating to force-feeding under the Mental Health Act 1983, Section 63.

> *B*, who was suffering from a borderline personality disorder coupled with post-traumatic stress disorder, was admitted under Section 3 of the Mental Health Act 1983 due to her irresistible urge to inflict self-harm. Whilst in hospital she began to refuse food as a method of inflicting self-harm. She was subsequently force-fed using a naso-gastric tube, but sought an injunction against this.

Thorpe J held that tube feeding did constitute treatment for *B*'s mental disorder within the meaning of the Mental Health Act, as it was treatment for the starvation that was a direct consequence of her mental disorder. This view was further upheld at the Court of Appeal. Lord Justice Hoffmann stated:

> It would seem strange to me if a hospital could, without the patient's consent, give her treatment directed to alleviating a psychopathic disorder showing itself in suicidal tendencies, but not without such consent be able to treat the consequences of a suicide attempt.

He went on to state:

> Nursing and care concurrent with the core treatment or as a necessary prerequisite to such treatment or to prevent the patient from causing harm to himself or to alleviate the consequences of the disorder are, in my view, all capable of being ancillary to a treatment calculated to alleviate or prevent a deterioration of the psychopathic disorder.

This suggests therefore that treatment refusals by competent patients detained under the Mental Health Act 1983 may not be respected if the treatment relates even quite distantly to a component of their mental disorder. Their Lordships did advise however that without the existence of a core treatment, in this case psychoanalytical therapy, tube feeding would by itself have been unlawful, as would the very detention of the appellant (Keywood, 1995).

Although the consideration of the use of best interests principles was not an issue that was pertinent to the case of B, it would be applicable if the patient concerned lacked capacity. B apparently valued and pursued forms of physical harm, in this case self-starvation, over treatment that could restore her health, perhaps as a means of dealing with difficult emotions in the only way she knew how to. This unusual evaluation of self-harm could be understood as arising in the context of a mental disorder: borderline personality disorder. Moreover, her unusual value system could be seen as preventing her from weighing up the information relevant to the decision to accept or refuse treatment for the physical consequences of her self-harm. In other words, a patient detained under the MHA for treatment of a mental disorder would be entitled to physical treatments using best interests principles, if he or she lacked capacity to consent to such treatment. Furthermore, if a patient in the emergency department was found to lack capacity and to need treatment for the consequences of self-harm, in his or her best interests, then this treatment could be given under the provisions of the MCA 2005 even if the MHA did not apply. Nonetheless, it is important to remember the presumption of capacity for all adults, including those who self-harm. Research evidence shows that a significant proportion of people who present to the emergency department following self-harm do retain the capacity to make decisions about medical treatment, and, furthermore, that relatively simple interventions can be used to improve impaired decision-making capacity in those who initially fail the test laid out in the MCA (Jacob et al., 2005).

In conclusion, despite legal guidance in the form of the Mental Capacity Act 2005 and the Mental Health Act 1983, as amended in 2007, there remains ambiguity in the management of some individuals who either lack capacity and/or have a mental disorder, particularly when such individuals refuse treatments. It is therefore important that psychiatrists are confident of the general principles guiding the management of patients who need treatment under either mental health or mental capacity legislation but remain prepared to take advantage of the legal support systems available in difficult or controversial cases.

- Self-harm is a complex behaviour with multi-factorial aetiological triggers. Many acts of self-harm are not directly associated with suicidal intent. They are often an attempt to communicate with others, to secure help, or to obtain relief from a difficult and otherwise overwhelming situation or emotional state.
- It has been established in case law (e.g. by the case of B v. Croydon Health Authority) that treatment for mental disorder under the Mental Health Act can include treatment of the physical consequences of self-harm, which results from that.
- It is possible for someone to meet the criteria for treatment of their mental disorder under the Mental Health Act, even if they retain DMC.

References

Adults with Incapacity (Scotland) Act) (2000) London: HMSO.

Appleby, L. (2009) Letter to Royal College of Psychiatrists: Mental Health Act 1983 and the treatment of the physical consequences of self-harm. www.rcpsych.ac.uk/rollofhonour/rcpsychnews/. . ./applebyletter.aspx.

Bellhouse, J., Holland, A., Clare, I. C., et al. (2003) Capacity-based mental health legislation and its impact on clinical practice: 2) treatment in hospital. Journal of Mental Health Law, 24–37.

Carpenter, W. T., Jr, Gold, J. M., Lahti, A. C., et al. (2000) Decisional capacity for informed consent in schizophrenia research. *Archives of General Psychiatry*, 57(6), 533–538.

David, A., Hotopf, M., Moran, P., et al. (2010) Mentally disordered or lacking capacity? Lessons for management of serious deliberate self-harm. *British Medical Journal*, 7, 341, c4489.

Grisso, T. & Appelbaum, P. S. (1991) Mentally ill and non-mentally-ill patients' abilities to understand informed consent disclosures for medication: Preliminary data. *Law and Human Behaviour*, 15(4), 377–388.

Grisso, T. & Appelbaum, P. S. (1995) The MacArthur Treatment Competence Study. III: Abilities of patients to consent to psychiatric and medical treatments. *Law and Human Behaviour*, 19(2), 149–174.

Grisso, T., Appelbaum, P. S. & Hill-Fotouhi, C. (1997) The MacCAT-T: A clinical tool to assess patients' capacities to make treatment decisions. *Psychiatric Services*, 48(11), 1415–1419.

Gunn, M. (1994) The meaning of incapacity. *Medical Law Review*, 2, 8–29.

Hassan, T. B., MacNamara, A. F., Davy, A., et al. (1999) Lesson of the week: Managing patients with deliberate self-harm who refuse treatment in the accident and emergency department. *British Medical Journal*, 319(7202), 107–109.

Hawton, K., Fagg, J. & McKeown, S. P. (1989) Alcoholism, alcohol and attempted suicide. *Alcohol and Alcoholism*, 24(1), 3–9.

Herring, J. (2008) Entering the fog: On the borderlines of mental capacity. *Indiana Law Journal*, 83(4). Article 16.

In the estate of Park (1953) 2 All E.R.40.

Jacob, R., Clare, I. C., Holland, A., et al. (2005) Self-harm, capacity, and refusal of treatment: Implications for emergency medical practice – a prospective observational study. *Emergency Medical Journal*, 22(11), 799–802.

Kennedy, I. (1992) Consent to treatment: The capable person. In: *Doctors, Patients, and the Law* (ed. Dyer, C.), pp. 44–71. Oxford: Blackwell Scientific Publications.

Keywood, K. (1995) *B v. Croydon Health Authority 1994*, CA: Force-feeding the Hunger Striker under the Mental Health Act 1983. Current Legal Issues.

Larkin, G. L., Marco, C. A. & Abbott, J. T. (2001) Emergency determination of decision-making capacity: Balancing autonomy and beneficence in the emergency department. *Academic Emergency Medicine*, 8(3), 282–284.

Mackay, N. & Barrowclough, C. (2005) Accident and emergency staff's perceptions of deliberate self-harm: Attributions, emotions and willingness to help. *British Journal of Clinical Psychology*, 44(2), 255–267.

Marson, D. C., Chatterjee, A., Ingram, K., et al. (1996) Toward a neurological model of competency: Cognitive predictors of capacity to consent in Alzheimer's disease using three different legal standards. *Neurology*, 46(3), 666–672.

Mason, J. K. & Laurie, G. T. (2006) *Mason and McCall Smith's Law and Medical Ethics*. 7th edn. Oxford University Press. *(When referring to this book, I am specifically referring to chapters 1, 10 and 20, which are titled Medical Ethics and Medical Practice, Consent to Treatment, and Mental Health and Human Rights, respectively.)*

McLean, S. (2009) Living wills and refusing treatment: The Kerrie Wooltorton case. Wooltorton blogs.bmj.com/.../sheila-mclean-on-advance-directives-and-the-case-of-K-Wooltorton.

Mental Capacity Act (2005) London: HMSO.

Mental Capacity Act, Code of Practice (2007). www.dca.gov.uk/legal-policy/mental-capacity/mca-cp.pdf.

Mental Health Act (1983) London: HMSO.

NICE Guidelines. Self-harm (2004) The short-term physical and psychological management and secondary prevention of self-harm in primary and secondary care. CG16.

Owen, G. S., David, A. S., Richardson, G., et al. (2009) Mental capacity, diagnosis and insight. *Psychological Medicine*, 39, 1389–1398.

Raymont, V., Bingley, W., Buchananan, A., et al. (2004) Prevalence of mental incapacity in medical inpatients and associated risk factors: Cross-sectional study. *Lancet*, 16–22(364), 1421–1427.

Roth, L. H., Meisel, A. & Lidz, C. W. (1977) Tests of competency to consent to treatment. *American Journal of Psychiatry*, 134 (3), 279–284.

Szmukler, G. (2004) Mental health legislation is discriminating and stigmatising In: *Every Family in the Land* (ed. Crisp, A.), The Royal Society of Medicine Press.

Wong, J. G., Clare, I. C. H., Gunn, M. J., *et al.* (1999) Capacity to make health care decisions: Its importance in clinical practice. *Psychological Medicine*, 29(2), 437–446.

Wong, J. G., Clare, I. C. H., Holland, A. J., *et al.* (2000) The capacity of people with a 'mental disability' to make a health care decision. *Psychological Medicine*, 30 (2), 295–306.

Case law

A Local Authority v. *E (by her Litigation Friend the Official Solicitor)* [2012].

B v. *Croydon Health Authority* [1995] 1 All ER 683.

Re B (Adult: Refusal of Medical Treatment) [2002] EWHC 429 (Fam).

Re C (Adult: Refusal of Medical Treatment) [1994] 1 All ER 819.

Re F (Mental Patient: Sterilisation) [1990] 2 AC 1.

Re R [1991] 4 ALL ER 177 CA.

Re SB (A Patient: Capacity To Consent To Termination) [2013] EWCOP 1417.

St George Healthcare NHS Trust v. *S* [1993] 3 All ER 673.

Index